Out-Patient (OPD) Services in Hospitals

Principles & Guidelines

Out-Patient (OPD) Services in Hospitals

Principles & Guidelines

Dr. Mohd. Faisal Khan
MBBS, PGDHM (IIHMR), AMAHA
Faculty (Health Management), Department of Management Studies,
Faculty of Management Studies and Information Technology (FMSIT),
Jamia Hamdard (Hamdard University), New Delhi, India
Formerly Medical Superintendent, H.L. Hospital, Aligarh
Medical Superintendent, S.S. Hospital, Moradabad
Senior Research Fellow, J.N. Medical College, Aligarh

Dr. Humera Khan
MBBS, MD
Formerly Senior Resident, J.N. Medical College, Aligarh

CBS

CBS Publishers & Distributors Pvt. Ltd.

New Delhi • Bengaluru • Chennai • Kochi • Kolkata • Mumbai
Hyderabad • Uttarakhand • Nagpur • Patna • Pune • Jharkhand

ISBN: 81-239-1337-0

First Edition: 2006
Reprint: 2019

Published by **Satish Kumar Jain** and produced by **Varun Jain** for
CBS Publishers & Distributors Pvt. Ltd.,
4819/XI Prahlad Street, 24 Ansari Road, Daryaganj, New Delhi - 110002
delhi@cbspd.com, cbspubs@airtelmail.in • www.cbspd.com
Ph.: 23289259, 23266861, 23266867 • Fax: 011-23243014

Corporate Office: 204 FIE, Industrial Area, Patparganj, Delhi - 110 092
Ph: 49344934 • Fax: 011-49344935
E-mail: publishing@cbspd.com • publicity@cbspd.com

Branches:

- ***Bengaluru:*** 2975, 17th Cross, K.R. Road, Bansankari 2nd Stage, Bengaluru - 70 • Ph: +91-80-26771678/79 • Fax: +91-80-26771680 E-mail: cbsbng@gmail.com, bangalore@cbspd.com
- ***Chennai:*** No. 7, Subbaraya Street, Shenoy Nagar, Chennai - 600030 Ph: +91-44-26681266, 26680620 • Fax: +91-44-42032115 E-mail: chennai@cbspd.com
- ***Kochi:*** Ashana House, 39/1904, A.M. Thomas Road, Valanjambalam, Ernakulum, Kochi • Ph: +91-484-4059061-65 Fax: +91-484-4059065 • E-mail: cochin@cbspd.com
- ***Kolkata:*** 6-B, Ground Floor, Rameshwar Shaw Road, Kolkata - 700014 Ph: +91-33-22891126/7/8 • E-mail: kolkata@cbspd.com
- ***Mumbai:*** 83-C, Dr. E. Moses Road, Worli, Mumbai - 400018 Ph: +91-9833017933, 022-24902340/41 • E-mail: mumbai@cbspd.com

Representatives:

- Hyderabad: 0-9885175004
- Patna: 0-9334159340
- Jharkhand: 0-9811541605
- Nagpur: 0-9021734563
- Pune: 0-9623451994
- Uttarakhand: 0-9716462459

Printed at:
India Binding House, Noida, UP (India)

Preface

The Out-Patient Department (OPD) is described as the hospital's "*shop window*". It is the first point of contact between the hospital and the community. The OPD facilities provide the main linkage of the hospital with the community. The OPD interacts with the neighbourhood and efficient out-patient services produce a favourable public image. When ambulatory care is given at premises that are part of a hospital, it is termed as "**Out-Patient Care**" and the services rendering or organizing it are called "**Out-Patient Services**". The area where these services are delivered is known as "**Out-Patient Department (OPD)**". The patient who visits OPD or Emergency Department is known as "Out-Patient (OP)". The Out-Patient Department is one of the growing points of the hospital mainly because there is shift in the centre of activities from in-patient (IP) towards out-patient (OP). The reason behind this shift is the rising cost of IP care and relative shortage of hospital beds with respect to needs. Out-patient department of hospital can be the *starting point* of quality of medical care provided to the patient's. Good OPD care can reduce the load on in-patient department (IPD) of the hospital. For some patients the OPD will be their first introduction to a hospital and many will be *nervous* and need *reassurance*. It is important that the atmosphere should be *welcoming, comfortable* and *humane*. Efficient and effective organization of OPD by competent health care professionals is essential for any hospital delivering out-patient services to the community. An attempt has been made to create a comprehensive profile of Out-Patient (OPD) Services in hospitals.

AUTHORS

Contents

Chapterization

Out-Patient (OPD) Services in Hospitals
Principles and Guidelines

1

Introduction

OVERVIEW

Ambulatory Care is the medical care provided to the patients who are not confined to bed. When such care is given at premises that are part of a hospital, it is termed as "**Out-Patient Care**" and the services rendering or organizing it are called "**Out-Patient Services**". The area where these services are rendered is called "**Out-Patient Department (OPD)**" (Goel and Kumar, 1984). "**Out-Patient (OP)**" is the one who visits OPD or Emergency Department (Pandey, 1990-1992).

Out-Patient Department (OPD) is *defined* "as a part of the hospital with allotted physical facilities and medical and other staff in sufficient numbers, with regularly schduled hours, to provide care for patients who are not registered as inpatients" (Sakharkar, 1999).

The Out-Patient Department (OPD) is described as the hospital's "**shop window**". It is the first point of contact between the hospital and the community. The Out-Patient Department (OPD) facilities provide the main linkage of the hospital with the community. The OPD interacts with the neighbourhood. Efficient out-patient services produce a favourable public image. The out-patients are becoming more and more important. The community gets the first impression of the hospital from the OPD. The reputation of the hospital can be made or marred by its impression upon the patient in the very first minutes of arrival at the hospital. Ambulatory care reduces dislocation of work, is cheaper and at the same time gives access to the various investigative and diagnostic facilities of the hospital. Patient's satisfaction with the hospital *OP services* is an important factor in influencing patient patronage and loyalty.

The Out-Patient Department is one of the growing points of the hospital mainly because there is shift in the centre of activities from *in-patient (IP)* towards *out- patient (OP)*. The reason behind this shift is the rising cost of IP care and relative shortage of hospital beds with respect to needs (Ghei, 1990). The shortage of hospital beds in Indian scenario is reflected in the data produced by Indian Economy Statistical Yearbook (1996) that 0.97 bed is shared by thousand Indians. Another reason for this shift is the immense development in the field of health care that has made it possible to treat a greater proportion of patients on the OP basis and reduce morbidity and mortality. Out-Patient (OP) treatment helps in avoiding disruption of family life that is an invariable accompaniment of In-Patient (IP) care (Agrawal, 1989).

WHO (WORLD HEALTH ORGANISATION) DEFINITION OF HOSPITAL

***A Hospital** is an integral part of a Social and Medical organization, the function of which is to provide for the population complete health care, both curative and preventive, and whose outpatient services reach out to the family and its home environment; the hospital is also a centre for the training of health workers and bio-social research.*

HEALTH AND HEALTHCARE SERVICES

Health is a fundamental human right. This implies that the state has a responsibility for the health of its people. National Governments all over the world are trying to expand and improve their healthcare services for the community. The healthcare services in developing countries are far from satisfactory and about 80 per cent of the population lives in rural areas and is deprived or have no access to modern medical and healthcare facilities. This leads to high rates of morbidity and mortality from a large number of diseases, which are curable and or otherwise preventable.

Healthcare services are designed to meet the health needs of the community through the use of available knowledge and resources. The healthcare services are delivered by the "**health system**", which includes the management sector and involves organizational matters. The main purpose of healthcare services is to improve the health status of the population. The targets to be achieved by healthcare services are:

- Mortality and morbidity reduction in the community
- An increase in life expectancy of the people
- Nutritional status of the community is to be improved
- Decrease in population growth rate
- Adequate provision of basic sanitation and hygienic conditions to the population
- Health manpower requirements and resources development

In India healthcare delivery systems includes:

- **Public Healthcare Delivery System** (Primary health centers, Sub-centres, Community health centers, Rural hospitals, District hospitals, Specialist hospitals, Teaching hospitals) funded and managed by the Government.
- **Private Healthcare Delivery System** (Private hospitals, Polyclinics, Nursing homes, Dispensaries) funded and managed by corporate sector.

Individuals are contributing in healthcare delivery to the community as General Practitioners and Clinicians (Park, K. 2000).

Health consultants are of the opinion that the problems in meeting the health needs of the population are mainly dependent on the capabilities to design and manage the healthcare delivery system *efficiently* and *effectively*.

Presently the healthcare delivery management systems are not operating well as unskilled persons are mainly managing them. There is a need to improve the functioning of healthcare management with the help of modern management tools in order to deliver quality healthcare services to the community.

MAGNITUDE AND IMPORTANCE OF OUT-PATIENT DEPARTMENT (OPD)

According to currently available statistics:

> "For each hospital bed, about 500 out-patients per year are given service. This implies that over 30 crore out-patients in a year are treated in the out-patient department of hospitals" (Sakharkar, 1999).

Importance of the Out-Patient Department lies in the following:

- An out-patient is the patient's first point of contact with the hospital and entry point into the health care delivery system.
- It is an inseparable link in the hierarchical chain of health care facilities.
- It contributes to reduction in morbidity and mortality.
- It helps in health promotion and disease prevention.
- It helps to reduce the number of admission to in-patient wards, thus, conserving scarce beds.
- It acts as a filter for in-patient admission, ensuring that only those patients are admitted who are most likely to benefit from in-patient care.
- It is the "shop window" of the hospital (Sakharkar,1999).

The Out-Patient Department (OPD) is needed to perform the following *main functions*:

- to diagnose and treat patients at an early stage,
- follow up treatment after discharge from the hospital, and
- to institute health education programme to educate the public in environmental hygiene (Indian Standard, 1986).

The out-patient department of a *general hospital* should have the following:

- General facilities
- Clinics of various medical discipline
- Support services like laboratories

- Pharmacy
- Blood Bank (Indian Standard, 1986)

OBJECTIVE AND SCOPE OF SERVICES

1. **Provision of general medical services to out-patients on scheduled/unscheduled basis:**
    - Preventive and promotive services (immunisation, screening, antenatal clinics, well baby clinics)
    - Curative (consultation, investigations, therapeutic procedures, speciality services)
    - Follow-up of discharged patients, chronic illnesses, post natal clinics, and
    - Rehabilitative (physiotherapy, occupational therapy; prosthetics and Orthotics).
2. **Family Welfare Services**; counselling
3. **Health Education**
4. **Medical, Nursing and Paramedical Education.**

LOCATION OF OUT-PATIENT DEPARTMENT (OPD)

1. Near the main roads and close to main hospital entrance, but with sufficient space to provide for parking etc., and to prevent noise and dust pollution.
2. Separate from in-patient wards and other departments, but connected with them:
    - Can function more efficiently in terms of scheduling and communications.
    - Easier for patients to find their way around.
    - Less patient and attendant traffic through central hospital.
    - Kept close when not in use.
    - Easier to expand, should a need arise.
3. Disadvantages of physically separate Out-patient and In-patient Departments:
    - Certain specialised diagnostic facilities may be available only in the in-patient section of the respective speciality thus causing inconvenience to the patients.

- Some out-patient facilities are required for use also by in-patients.
- A separate facility may require duplication of certain services that could otherwise be shared, specially; satellite laboratories.
- Distance between in-patient and out-patient facilities may inconvenience the doctors who have the responsibilities in both areas.

4. OPD should be close to:
   - Medical Records
   - Laboratory
   - Radiology
   - Pharmacy

   It should be adjacent to Casualty/Emergency Department.
5. Preferable to have OPD of all specialities in same building to facilitate cross-references between various specialities.
6. The Out-Patient Department (OPD) should be located close to the main entrance with independent approach and should be segregated from the In-Patient Department (IPD) so that patients visiting the Out-Patient Department need not pass through the In-Patient Department. Some of the treatment facilities like radiology, pathology, physiotherapy and blood bank should be interposed between OPD and IPD so as to be equally accessible to both OPD and IPD.

OPD Clinics such as *antenatal*, *gynaecology* and sometimes *paediatrics* also share equipment with their counterparts in respective in-patient wards.

The size of the OPD depends upon the volume of attendance, the clinics provided and the extent of other facilities, like laboratory, blood bank, health education programme, operating facilities, emergency wards, etc. (Indian Standard, 1986).

Recommended size of OPD is 2 - 3 square feet per OPD attendance.

PHYSICAL FACILITIES IN THE OUT-PATIENT DEPARTMENT (OPD)

The OPD's may be a *horizontal spread* or *vertical*. In vertically placed OPD's, consideration must be given for adequate provision of vertical transport, not only in the form of lift but also ramps in addition to the usual stairs. There can be the use of escalators in the future.

Each clinic in the OPD must be twin room. The outer room where the patient comes in contact with the Doctor and the inner room where the patient is examined. The twin rooms of the OPD should be sandwiched between two corridors. The outer corridor used for entry and exit of patients, while the rear corridor used to provide services to the OPD's. Each consultation chamber will need a table for doctor, chairs, patients stool, wash basin, examination couch, X-Ray view box, foot step and other equipment as required for each speciality.

Facilities in OPD Wing

The OPD wing will have the following facilities:

Entrance Lobby

- Patients and attendants will wait here prior to registration and proceeding for examination.
- This area should have sinages adequately displaying how the patient is to proceed.
- This area should also have display boards providing, relevant information.
- Waiting time of patient's and attendants could be gainfully used by providing educational programmes.
- Adequate toilet facilities should be provided close to this area.

Reception, Registration, Cash Counter and Information

- Patients coming for consultation will be registered before they proceed towards the consultation chamber.
- They will need to deposit cash for registration, investigations and for other purposes.
- A number of patients need information regarding the facilities and how to proceed.

Sub-waiting spaces

- After registration, patients will proceed to the doctor's clinics.
- They will need to wait till the doctor calls them.
- Serious patients could be called out of turn, or may be advised to attend emergency instead.

- Waiting space for *eye* patients should be planned *away* from direct sunlight while that of paediatric should have suitable space for children.

Consultation Rooms (Doctors clinics)

Requirement of each clinic will vary with the speciality and the quantum of work.

Clinics requiring special consideration are as under:

Orthopaedics clinic

This will require facility for examination of fracture patient's and for plaster application. A number of patients may be brought on wheelchair or trolley. Accordingly adequate movement space should be provided.

Eye clinic

The room where vision testing is done should have a minimum length of 6 metres. However, by placing a mirror, the length could be brought down to 3 metres. Provision of making the room dark will be needed where the patient is being examined.

ENT clinic

ENT clinic will need an audiometry room. The room will require to be made sound proof.

Dental clinic

This clinic will require a dental lab for making Dentures and other dental items. Facility for water will be required. The dental chair will require provision for water inlet, water outlet and electricity. A small dark room for processing dental X-Ray films will be required.

Gynaecology and Obstetric clinic

Patients will need to pass urine prior to examination. Necessary facility of toilet will be needed either in the clinic or close by.

Paediatric clinic

Facility will be required where the weight and height of the child could be taken. Facility will also be required to give immunisation to children.

Psychiatry clinic

The clinic will require dado till 4 feet height. Electrical fittings should be protected. Facility for carrying out ECT will be required.

OPD in addition will, require an injection room, treatment room and an ECG room.

IMPROVING THE OUT-PATIENT DEPARTMENT (OPD)

- Analyze the diagnoses of the patients attending, find their six main diseases.
- Determine the simplest, cheapest and most effective routine for treating these diseases.
- Teach auxillaries how to diagnose and treat these diseases.
- Pay more attention to more serious conditions, which they must learn to distinguish from them.
- Provide the necessary equipment, rubber stamps, prepacked drugs, stationary, etc., and sufficient of the simple things like dressing forceps.
- Trace the flow of patients through the hospital complex. Can it be rationalized by simple work services such as the alteration of doors etc.
- Examine the queues that form. Identify the cause of delays. Can these be removed by altering the disposition of staff etc.
- Where relevant let the auxilliaries listen in on your consultations with the referred patients, so that they may learn continually (Kumar, 2000).

INDIAN SCENARIO OF OUT-PATIENT DEPARTMENT (OPD)

In the Indian scenario we find that 2-3 attendants usually accompany each patient. Accordingly provision of services like toilets, drinking water facility, waiting space, etc. should be made for twice or thrice the number.

In India, OPD's are generally overcrowded and cater for a much higher number of patients than were originally planned for. This leads to the patient dis-satisfaction due to long waiting queues, overcrowding, lack of of adequate provision of services and lack of acceptable behaviour of staff (Chaskar,[1996], Ghosh, [1990], Ratnam [1995] and Satyanarayan, *et.al* [1994])

The hospitals OPD's are generally overcrowded and cater for a much higher number of patients than were originally planned for. The OPD's should, therefore, be planned for *maximum utilisation, quick turn over, less waiting time* for the patient and the *minimum number* of *queues*. In overcrowded OPD's especially of large hospitals, screening of patients can be done either through general duty officer or through referral polyclinic's to save the time of the consultants. The referral polyclinic may be either a part of the hospital complex itself or may be in the form of a satellite polyclinic in the catchment area.

PATIENT FLOW PATTERN IN OUT-PATIENT DEPARTMENT (OPD)

Patient flow in OPD usually progresses from enquiry and registration to waiting then to examination rooms and then to investigation facilities and finally the pharmacy (Sakharkar, 1999). The flow chart of activities and movements in the OPD is given in figure 1.1.

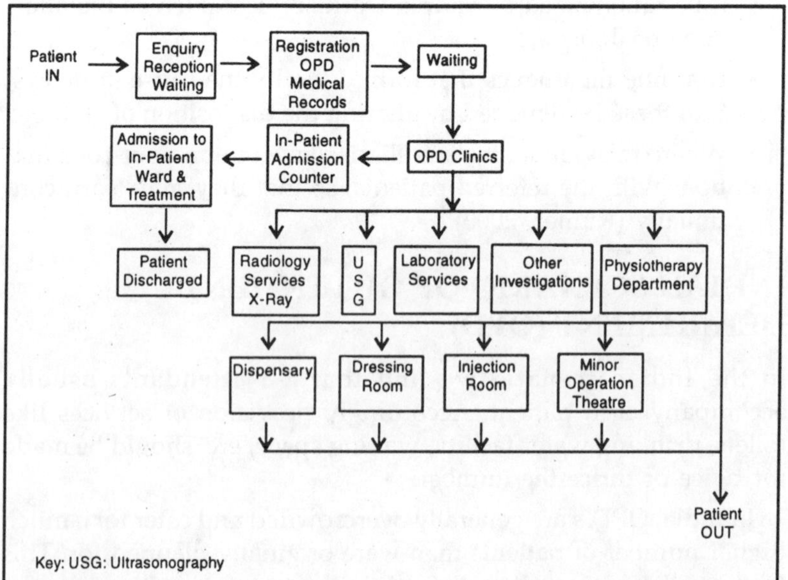

Fig. 1.1: Patient Flow Chart of Out-Patient Department (OPD)

QUALITY IN OUT-PATIENT DEPARTMENT (OPD)

Quality is an important multi-dimensional attribute of health care. Many health services researchers and providers focus on whether the care that is provided is *evidence-based.* Economists typically view quality as a component of non-price competition. Quality is defined as "the degree to which health services for individuals and populations increase the likelihood of desired health outcomes and are consistent with current professional knowledge. According to the Agency for Healthcare Research and Quality (AHRQ) quality health care is "doing the right thing at the right time in the right way for the right person and having the best result possible". Regulators and most academic commentators have historically employed a three-part framework (*structure, process,* and *outcome*) to assess quality of care. Some consumers may focus on how long they must wait for an appointment, and how they are treated when they arrive at the provider's office. Depending on which of these attributes is emphasized and the particular condition being evaluated, it is possible for the same care to be simultaneously deemed high quality and low quality.

Many health care providers and health services researchers view quality as effectively binary: a provider is either delivering high quality care to a particular patient or he is not doing so. This paradigm treats the resources of the individual consumer as immaterial to the determination of whether the care is of acceptable quality. Conversely, economists and legal scholars sometimes treat quality as an attribute that can be traded-off against price and other attributes of health care.

Health care quality actually encompasses many distinct factors, and the delivery system must perform well on each factor if it is to provide high quality care. These factors include whether the medical diagnosis is correct, whether the "right" treatment is selected (with the "right" treatment varying, depending on the underlying diagnosis and patient preferences and resources), whether the treatment is performed in a technically competent manner, whether service quality is adequate, and whether patients are able to access the care they desire without undue travel and inconvenience. Whether cutting edge technology and treatments are available is a component of health care quality, but it is not the only consideration. Information is necessary for consumers to make decisions about the care they will receive, and determine whether they are receiving the type of care they prefer and can afford (www.usdoj.gov).

Out-patient department of hospital can be the *starting point* of quality of medical care provided to the patient's. Good OPD care can reduce the load on-inpatient. Operational aspects of OPD such as hour and timing of OPD, staff deployed in the unit to deal with the load of the patient and queuing time should be continuously monitored so as to ensure continuous improvement in the quality of services offered by the unit (Goel and Kumar, 2004).

MANAGEMENT

Management is defined "As the art of creating a fine climate for work in a group enterprise (through the performance of managerial functions); so that people working therein can give their maximum contribution towards the attainment of common objectives" (Gupta, 2003). It is the process whereby resources are utilized in a most effective and efficient manner in order to attain the objectives of the institution.

- **Effectiveness** is the degree of attainment of predetermined objectives and targets of a programme. If a hospital decided to admit and provide medical care to all surgery cases and it could treat only 50 per cent of such cases then it is 50 per cent effective.
- **Efficiency** is the relationship between the results obtained and the resources utilized in obtaining the results of the organization. If a hospital has made huge investment on the infrastructure, manpower and equipment designed to manage critical and specialized cases but is managing minor ailments only then the hospital is not efficient.

Functions Constituting Managerial Activity

As identified by Tripathi and Reddy (1997) functions constituting managerial activity are as follows:

- Planning
- Organizing
- Directing
- Controlling

Planning – It is a continuous process of selecting and developing best course of action to accomplish objectives. It is the function that determines in advance what should be done. It is required to be done whenever a new hospital or programme or activity is to be initiated. It may also be required while managing a major problem in the existing institution. In a hospital, the decision of whether the dispensary should be managed and established by the hospital or be given on contract should be taken based on the SWOT (strengths, weaknesses, opportunities and threats) analysis. The process of selection is based on the strengths, weakness of the organization and the opportunities and threats in the environment. The administrator must analyze availability of required expertise, finances, regular supply of drugs etc. He may also have to consider availability of contractors in the region, cost factor involved and chances of interruptions in the delivery of services by the contractor.

According to Chandler, Jr. A. D. (1962) "Strategy can be defined as the determination of basic long term goals and objectives of an enterprise and the adoption of courses of action and the allocation of resources for carrying out these goals".

Components of strategy are:

- Purpose and mission,
- Objectives and goals and
- Policies and programme strategies (Srinivasan, 2002).

Whenever there are a number of ways of sorting a problem, the process of selection of best one is known as strategic planning. Strategic planning involves deciding what the major goals of the entire institution will be and what policies will guide the institution in its pursuits of these goals.

Organizing - It is an orderly manner of bringing together and coordinating all human and physical resources. It is setting up the framework or apparatus and making it possible for groups to do the work. Healthcare delivery organization, involves the systematizing of all technical, administrative and related activities and personnel so as to lead to satisfaction to patients, employees and the agencies that make it possible to operate.

The process of organizing consists of:

- Developing an orderly structure
  - Different functions to be performed in the institution
  - Work to be performed by one person

- Human resource requirement
- Physical resource requirement
- Grouping and coordinating the functions

- Delineating relationships
  - Assigning responsibility and authority
  - Fixing accountability

Directing – After plans have been made and the institution has been established and staffed, the next sequence of event is to move towards its defined objectives through proper directing. "Directing is the interpersonal aspect of managing by which subordinates are led to understand and contribute effectively and efficiently to the attainment of enterprise objectives" (Koontz and O' Donnell, 1972).

Directing involves three sub functions:

- Communication – It is an instrument of direction. It is through communication that the superior gives orders, allocates jobs, explains duties and assures performance. Efficient communication is a two-way process.
- Leadership – The success of every institution is dependent upon the quality of its leadership. "Leadership is the lifting of man's visions to higher sights, the raising of man's performance to a higher standard, the building of man's personality beyond its normal limitations" (Drucker, 1970).
- Motivation – It is the process of channeling a person's inner drives so that he wants to accomplish the goals of the institution.

Controlling – It is checking to make sure the work is progressing satisfactorily. "Controlling is determining what is being accomplished, that is, evaluating the performance and if necessary, applying corrective measures so that the performance takes place according to plans" (Terry, 1968).

Control process involves the following steps:

- Establishing standards of performance.
- Measuring current performance and comparing it against the established standards.
- Taking action to correct any performance that does not meet those standards.

CONCLUSION

Out-Patient Department (OPD) is the point of contact between the hospital and the community. It is the patient's first point of contact with the hospital and entry point into the health care delivery system. The Out-Patient Department (OPD) is described as the hospital's "*shop window*". The community gets the first impression of the hospital from the OPD. Many patients gain their impression of the hospital from the OPD. Hospital could do much to convey a favourable impression to the patient at this point. Patient's satisfaction with the hospital **Out-Patient** services is an important factor in influencing patient patronage and loyalty. Recent years have seen a change of trend from hospitalization towards ambulatory treatment. Not only does this cut down on the cost of treatment but also helps in avoiding disruption of family life, which is an invariable accompaniment of hospitalization. With the recent concept of *day care services* the incidence of hospitalization can be brought down still further.

REFERENCES

1. Agrawal, A.K. *Planning and Organization of Ambulatory Care*, Journal of Hospital Administration, 7(1):38-43, 1989.
2. Agrawal, A.N. and Verma, H.O. *Indian Economy Statistical Yearbook*, 274, 1996.
3. Chandler, Jr. A.D. *Strategy and Structure*, Cambridge (Mass): MIT Press,1962.
4. Chaskar, R.P. *Study of Satisfaction Levels of Patients Visiting Charak Hospital*, Indore, Journal of Hospital Administration 34(3&4): 198-205, 1996.
5. Drucker, P. *Practice of Management*, Allied Publishers Pvt. Ltd., New Delhi, 1970.
6. Ghei, P.N. *Selected Readings in Hospital Administration*, 1990.
7. Ghosh, B.N. *A Case Study of Management of the Outpatient System in a Health Centre*, Indian Society of Health Administrators 22-24(1): 28-32, 1990.
8. Goel, S.L. and Kumar, R. *Out-Patient Department Hospital Administration and Management*, 2:34-37, 1984.
9. Goel, S.L. and Kumar, R. *Hospital Supportive Services*, Deep & Deep Publications PVT. LTD., New Delhi, 2004.
10. Gupta, R. N. *A Textbook of Business Studies*,: S. Chand & Company Ltd., New Delhi, 2003.

11. Indian Standard; *Recommendations for Basic requirements of General Hospital Buildings,* Part 2, Indian Standard Institutions, New Delhi, 1986.
12. Koontz, H. D. and O'Donnell, Cyril, J. *Principles of Management-An Analysis of Managerial Functions,* McGraw-Hill Kogakusha Ltd. 5th ed., Tokyo, 1972.
13. Kumar, A. *Encyclopaedia Of Hospital Administration And Development,* Volume 2, Institute For Sustainable Development Lucknow & Anmol Publications PVT.LTD., New Delhi, 2000.
14. Pandey, Dr. Ranjit *Readings in Hospital Management,* 1990-1992.
15. Park, K. *Parks Textbook of Preventive and Social Medicine,* M/s Banarsidas Bhanot Publishers, Jabalpur, 2000.
16. Ratnam, A. V. *A Study of Socio Economic Conditions and Satisfaction Levels of Patients Visiting a Corporate Hospital,* Journal of Hospital Administration 32(3&4): 129-54, 1995.
17. Sakharkar, B.M. *Principles of Hospital Administration and Planning,* Jaypee Brothers Medical Publishers (P) Ltd., New Delhi 1999.
18. Satyanarayan, N., *et al. A Study of Four Major Areas in Out-Patient Department of NIMS Special Reference to Patient Satisfaction,* Journal of Hospital Administration 31(3&4):173-181, 1994.
19. Srinivasan, R. *Strategic Management the Indian Context,* Prentice-Hall of India Private Limited, New Delhi, 2002.
20. Terry, R. G. *Principles of Management*: Richard D. Irwin., Homewood, III, 1968.
21. Tripathi, P. C. and Reddy, P. N. *Principles of Management,* Tata McGraw-Hill Publishing Company Limited, New Delhi 1997.
22. Website:http://www.usdoj.gov/atr/public/health_care/204694/chapter1.htm.

2

Out-Patient Department (OPD) in a Multidisciplinary Hospital

- ★ Overview
- ★ Terminology
- ★ Hospital Profile
- ★ The Existing System of Out-Patient Department (OPD)
- ★ Discussion
- ★ Recommendations
- ★ Conclusion
- ★ References

OVERVIEW

Hospital is a phenomenon of 20th century. Its evolution of supporting sick from normal to care of sick and now it is sophistication of providing preventive, promotive, curative and rehabilitative services is phenomenal. As the hospital has grown in stature, so has its important arm, out-patient department. The activities of out-patient departments have made the hospital a real force in the community programme, for the prevention of diseases. Much of the investigations and diagnostic work that formerly required admission to hospital wards can now be carried out in a well-equipped out-patient department. The concept of **"extended ambulatory services"** is borne out of the fact that certain diseases are treated right in out-patient department, without getting patients admitted for long durations as in-patients, thus, reducing expenses for the patients, community and exchequer. Out-patient department services are corollary to in-patient services in the form of general out-patient department, day care, home-care and rehabilitative centres. It is important for hospital and health care planners to know about the catchment area of the hospital so that cost-effective and cost containment techniques will be employed before hospital gets commissioned. This is particularly true, when tremendous strides have been made as far as patients care through out-patient department is concerned (Ahmad, R., Tabish, S. A., Qadiri, G. J. and Mustafa, A., 2001).

The primary function of a hospital is rendering quality patient care. The patient is the ultimate consumer to the hospital. It is one of the yardstick to measure the success of service that it produces. The effectiveness of the hospital relates to provision of good patient care as intended. The *patient satisfaction* is the real testimony to the efficiency of hospital management. Since the hospital serves all the members of the society the expectations of the users differ from one individual to another individual because everyone carries a particular set of thoughts, feelings and needs. Hence, determination of patient's real feelings is very difficult. Satisfaction is an important element in the evaluation stage. It refers to the consumer's state of being adequately rewarded. Adequacy of satisfaction is a result of matching the actual past experience with the expected reward. Patients form certain expectations prior to the visit to the hospital. Once patients come to the hospital and experience the facilities by themselves, they may then become either satisfied or dissatisfied. Satisfaction or dissatisfaction refers to emotional response to the evaluation of service, consumption and experience. It will have *five key elements*.

They are:

1. **Expectations**
2. **Performance**
3. **Comparison**
4. **Confirmation/Disconfirmation**
5. **Discrepancy**

Factors Influencing Patient Satisfaction

There are five determinants of patient satisfaction, they are:

1. **Reliability:** The ability to perform promised service dependably and accurately.

2. **Responsiveness:** The willingness to help the patients and provide prompt service.
3. **Assurance:** The knowledge and courtesy of employees and their ability to convey trust and confidence.
4. **Empathy:** The provision of caring and individualized attention to patients.
5. **Tangibles:** The appearance of physical facilities, equipment, personal and communication materials.

Excellently managed hospitals are having the following practices:

1. Top service hospitals are patient obsessed. They have a clear sense of their target customers and their needs.
2. The best service hospitals set high service quality standards. The standards must be set appropriately high, which leads to patient satisfaction.
3. Culture, subculture and social classes are important in determining the satisfaction levels. Culture is the fundamental determinant of an individuals wants and behaviour. It refers to a set of feelings of the patient or his relatives. Social class reflects sex, income, occupation, education, area of residence and recreational preferences, etc. which are important in determining the satisfaction levels.
4. The patients behaviour is greatly influenced by social factors like reference groups, ideas and beliefs. Reference groups here refer to peers, relatives, neighbours and friends. The family members are the important persons in influencing the patient.
5. The persons satisfaction is influenced by the psychological factors such as perception, learning and attitudes.

Apart from the above, other factors that influences the patient satisfaction include:

- Availability of adequate staff
- Availability of physical facilities and equipment
- Design of the unit
- Cleanliness
- Environment
- Availability of clinical services
- Work load of the staff

- Behaviour of the doctors, nursing staff and paramedical staff
- Effectiveness of management functions
- Leadership styles of administrators
- Communication channels, policies and procedures

Perceptions of the out-patients towards *Registration Procedure* can be studied by analyzing the following parameters:

- Reception services are good (Yes/No)
- Adequate information is available at reception counter (Yes/No)
- Time spent at registration counter is satisfactory (Yes/No)
- Present system at registration counter is satisfactory (Yes/No)
- Counters provided for registration are enough (Yes/No)
- On the whole registration procedure is good (Yes/No)
- There is need of security staff at registration counters (Yes/No) (Sreenivas , T. and Prasad, G., 2003)

The basic function of the out-patient department is to diagnose and to treat home-based patients and if needed accept them as in-patients. A good deal of the diagnostic and treatment accommodation can be of a general nature used at different clinic sessions by different, specialists. Too much separate accommodation for specialisms is wasteful, for much of it will be underused most of the time.

For some patients the department will be their first introduction to a hospital and many will be *nervous* and need *reassurance*. It is important that the atmosphere should be welcoming, comfortable and humane. The department should be so located so that it is easily reached by both the walking public and vehicles. A separate entrance is desirable and this should not be located too near the reception point for ambulances and for accident cases or the mortuary. Out-patients should not have to pass through any other part of the hospital to reach the department. It is an advantage if the department can be entirely at *street level* as some patients may find movement difficult.

In an out-patient department, the patient visits the doctor, normally on his own, initiative, to obtain help or treatment for a personal problem or ailment The advantage of treating the patient in the out-patient department is that it *eliminates* the need for or *reduces* length of hospitalization and consequently the cost to the patient. There may also be clinic sessions attended by numbers of people and organized for a particular purpose, such as immunization. In this it is similar to a health center, but the diagnostic techniques and treatment are more sophisticated. The *sequence* for patients is *reception, registration, waiting* and *consultation.* In some cases treatment or referral to another specialist department may be needed. Prescriptions may be collected at a dispensary on the way out. It is essential to have an enquiry or registration point at the entrance, associated with a general waiting space. Also sub-waiting spaces adjoining the clinic to which patient's are directed is desirable. These reduce the scale of the general waiting space and assist the flow of patient's through the department. The key to operational efficiency in the out-patient department is efficient patient flow. Patient's toilets and telephones should be provided and perhaps a refreshment counter, a shop and a children's playroom at the general waiting space.

Usually most of the consulting suites are general purpose, consisting either of ranges of combined consulting and examination rooms or of smaller consulting rooms with examination rooms adjoining. Some specialties may need rooms designed for a particular purpose. A clinical room is required for treatments such as dressings, a room for urine tests etc., clean and dirty utility rooms and a sisters office. An operating suite for minor conditions may be needed, together with day space and a day ward in which patient's can recover before going home. Although proximity is desirable, this operating suite need not be immediately adjoining the department.

The department needs easy access to the radio diagnostic facilities, medical records, to the dispensary and if possible to physiotherapy. Out-patients may have to visit any or all of these. Although these departments also serve the rest of the hospital it is an advantage if access to them can be as little associated as possible with the other main routes within the hospital. Proximity to the pathology laboratories is also desirable for the delivery of specimens (Health Facility Planning, 2000).

Out-patient services are the most important services provided by all the hospitals as it provides services to a large number of patients at a low cost. The patients suffering from diseases of minor, serious, acute and chronic nature are examined and clinically managed in OPD. In ordinary hospitals, the same doctor examines all categories of patients while in secondary and tertiary care hospitals, patients are examined by specialists. Efficient and effective management of OPD's by competent health care professionals can lighten the burden on the wards of the hospital (Goel and Kumar, 2004).

The number of people seeking out-patient care from hospitals would not matter so much if there were staff and facilities available in proportion to the demand. Most of the time, there are not, and competent doctors in particular are almost always critically scarce (Kumar, 2000).

The origin of ambulatory care visits can be determined by the same statistical methodology as that used for in-patients. Ambulatory care visits are usually found in a much smaller area than that for in-patients, but both primary and secondary areas should be identified (Hardy and Lammers, 1986).

TERMINOLOGY

Ambulatory Care: Out-patient care or services

Arrival Pattern: It is the study of the pattern in which patients arrive at the registration counter.

Patient Flow: It is the flow of patient from one service counter to another.

Queue Length: It is the number of patients waiting to receive service at given interval of time.

Response Time: It is the time taken to respond to a patient in order to provide service to that patient.

Service Time: This is the duration for which a doctor observes and then prescribes treatment to the patient.

Waiting Time: This is the duration for which a patient waits before receiving a service.

Work Flow: This is the manner in which work moves from one service counter to another service counter.

HOSPITAL PROFILE

The multidisciplinary hospital is a 250 bedded tertiary care hospital set up by X health care society and is located in the centre of the city. The institution became operational about a decade back. It has completed many years of successful running. It is financially supported by the society for developmental activities and advancement facilities. It runs on *"no-profit no-loss"* basis. More than ten percentages of patients reporting to the hospital are treated free on the recommendation of consultants.

The Mission of the hospital is

"To Serve All Sections Of The Society"

The Slogan of the hospital is

"The Hospital That Provides Quality Health Care"

The institution has made rapid progress within a very short period of time. It runs several different Out-Patient (OP) specialities and runs both the morning and the evening OPDs. The total out-patient attendance in the year 2003 was 105970 patients. The daily average OP attendance is 350 patients per day and at an average 40 per day admissions took place in the year 2003.

The commissioning of this tertiary care hospital in the state is considered as a major revolution, keeping in view the fact that the region has the highest incidence of a number of diseases and lacks behind in the availability of the treatment, in proportion to population and area. This institution was borne out of the dream to provide highest standards of quality health care to the people of the region and neighbouring states.

The catchment area of the hospital is not limited to city alone but extends to whole of the state as well as neighbouring states. It is one of the largest tertiary care hospital in the country and is managed by highly qualified, competent, experienced and dedicated clinical, paramedical and managerial staff. It is equipped with the latest health care technology.

This sprawling tertiary care hospital is centrally air-conditioned complex built at the cost of Rs. XY crores and is spread over an area of more than one lakh square feet. Equipped with the latest health care technology this health care hub aims to provide comprehensive health care of world-class standards and quality through highly competent dedicated team of health care professionals and latest medical technology.

The hospital offers state of art facilities ranging from preventive health care services to invasive and advanced interventional and surgical procedures. The hospital offers *single centre concept* where a patient can seek a complete range of investigation and therapeutic facilities. The hospital boosts of several operation theatres with the provision of laminar flow where all sort of surgeries such as a open and closed heart surgeries etc. can be performed.

There are intensive care areas, which include emergency, surgical and medical ICU's.

Emergency department is well equipped with all sophisticated medical equipments to treat any emergency reporting to the hospital.

The hospital has well equipped mobile cardiac care ambulance for the shifting of patients.

A 24-hour blood bank facility is available to meet the requirements of blood transfusion. In order that human blood is efficiently utilized the concept of blood components is promoted wherein the whole blood is separated into multiple units of blood components, which are finally transfused into different individuals with different needs. Apheresis facility wherein important components of the blood are removed and the remaining part is transfused back is also available in the blood bank.

Organizational Structure of the Hospital

The hospital has the following:

1. Chairman
2. Managing Director
3. Medical Superintendent
4. Deputy Medical Superintendent
5. Nursing Superintendent
6. Hospital Administrator
7. Consultants
8. Senior Residents
9. Junior Residents
10. Public Relation Officer
11. Personnel Officer
12. Chief Accounts Officer
13. Housekeeper
14. Security Incharge

15. Maintenance Incharge
16. Stores Incharge
17. Equipments Incharge
18. Library Incharge
19. Support Staff (Nursing, Sanitary, Paramedical, Administrative, etc.)

Organogram

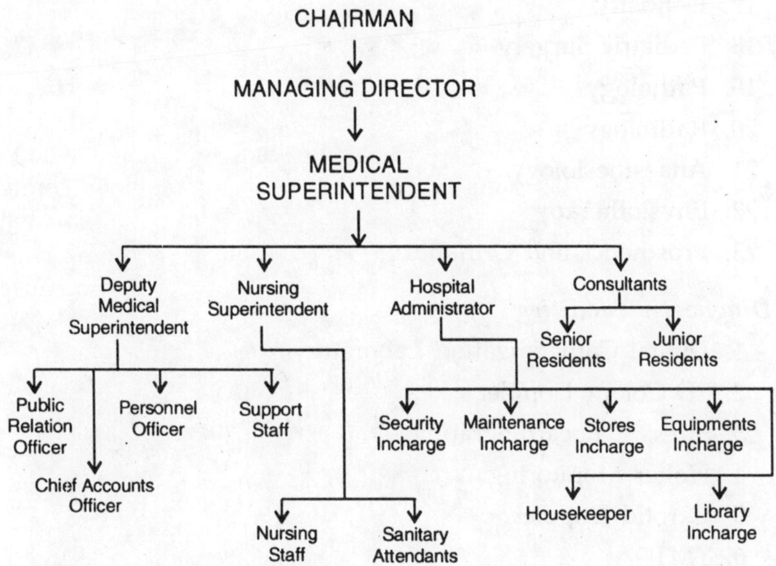

Facilities Provided by the Hospital

Specialities

1. General Medicine
2. General Surgery
3. Cardiology
4. Psychiatry
5. Dermatology
6. Neurology
7. Neurosurgery
8. Paediatrics

9. Gastroenterology
10. Nephrology and Dialysis
11. Orthopaedics
12. Urology
13. Opthalmology
14. Otorhinolaryngology
15. Obstetrics and Gynaecology
16. Cardiothoracic
17. Dentistry
18. Pediatric Surgery
19. Pathology
20. Radiology
21. Anaesthesiology
22. Physiotherapy
23. Prosthetics and Orthotics

Diagnostic Facilities

1. Digital Catheterization Laboratory
2. 2D Colour Doppler
3. Stress Echocardiography
4. Holter Monitoring
5. Carotid Doppler
6. TMT
7. ECG
8. PFT
9. EMG
10. Cine Angiography
11. Gastroscopy
12. Audiometry
13. Radiography
14. Sonography
15. Cystoscopy
16. Bronchoscopy
17. Laproscopy

18. Arthroscopy
19. CT Scan
20. Urodynamic Lab
21. Others

Support Services

1. Laboratory
2. Blood bank
3. Medical Records Unit
4. Ambulances
5. Maintenance Workshop
6. Photography Unit
7. Library
8. Computer Section
9. Others

THE EXISTING SYSTEM OF OUT-PATIENT DEPARTMENT (OPD)

OPD Organization Structure of the multidisciplinary hospital is:

1. Medical Superintendent
2. Deputy Medical Superintendent
3. Honorary Consultants
4. Senior Consultants
5. Junior Consultants
6. Senior Residents
7. Junior Residents
8. Nursing Superintendent
9. Nursing Incharge
10. Staff Nurses
11. Nursing Aide
12. OPD Attendant
13. Sanitary Staff

Hospital Policy of Patient Care in OPD's

- Patient has to pay registration charges before he can consult a doctor.
- Registration fee is valid for 5 days and the patient can visit the same consultant without paying any consultation fees again.
- When a patient reports for follow up after 5 days, then again he will have to pay the registration charges.
- In case of cross referral in OPD's within the hospital no extra charges are to be borne by the patient.
- Free patients are to be seen as per hospital rules.
- Medico Legal Cases (MLC) cases are to be seen.

Location

OPD's are located on 3 different floors of the leading multi-disciplinary hospital *viz.*:

1. **Ground Floor**
2. **First Floor**
3. **Basement**

Various OPD's in the Multidisciplinary Hospital

1. Cardiac Rehabilitation
2. Cardiology
3. Dental Surgery
4. Dermatology (Skin)
5. Dieatry
6. Endocrinology and Diabetes
7. ENT
8. Gastroenterology
9. General Medicine and Paediatrics
10. General Surgery and Urology
11. Nephrology
12. Neurology
13. Neurosurgery
14. Obstetrics and Gynaecology
15. Oncology

16. Opthalmology (Eye)
17. Orthopaedic Surgery
18. Paediatrics
19. Pain Clinic
20. Physiotherapy
21. Psychiatry
22. Urology

OPD is closed on Sunday

Physical Facilities

The main entrance of the hospital opens into the central lobby which has the following:

1. Enquiry Counter
2. Reception Counter
3. OPD Counter
4. Admission/Payments Counter
5. Waiting Space with Seating Arrangement
6. Toilets (separate for males and females)

Patient Flow

The patients whether new or old first reports at the enquiry and reception counter of the unit, than reports to OPD counter and then makes himself comfortable in the waiting space of the OPD's. Then patients are being called in respective OPD's according to their number in the queue. After being examined by consultant they are advised investigations and then again to report back to the OPD or they are simply advised treatment and issued a prescription or they are advised to avail services of injection room, dressing room, minor OT and pharmacy or they are advised to get admitted in the hospital if the condition so warrants.

Enquiry & Reception Counter

Located near the main entrance of the hospital and it is taken care of by two persons who have telephone facility.

Timings

9 A.M. - 1 P. M.

5 P. M. - 7 P. M.

The main functions performed is to release information about various OPD's such as their location to the patients and information regarding fees, availability of consultants etc. They also help the patients in filling up of various forms of the hospital.

Salient Observations

- Time spent at the enquiry counter was found normally acceptable to patients even if they spent more than 5-10 minutes.
- Patients accumulating during peak hours.
- Queue discipline not followed.
- Sufficient attention is not paid to clear the rush at or near the main entrance and the enquiry counter.
- Signboard is not placed at strategic position identifying the enquiry counter.
- Board displaying the location of various doctors is not available at reception.
- Staff behaviour at the reception is not acceptable to few patients.

OPD Counter

- Patient after filling the registration form reports at the OPD counter.
- Person sitting on the counter takes the form and out-patient card is made.
- Patients deposit fees.
- Entries are made in the computers installed at the counter.
- Computerised receipts and stickers bearing OPD numbers, name of the patient, age, sex, charges, address etc., are pasted over the *out-patient card* and the *patient's identity card.*
- Out-patient card and the patient's identity card are then handed over to the patients. Once the patient has shown to a particular consultant the out-patient card comes back to the OPD counter, which also acts as a Medical Records Section. For the follow up cases the patient's identity card is used to take out the out-patient card.
- The registration fees is Rs. 50/ which includes registration charges of Rs. 10/ and Rs. 40/ as consultation fees.

- The *colour* of the out-patient card changes every year, and the colour of the staff card is blue. If the patient has to be admitted, then he will have to deposit money on the IPD counter i.e. Admission and Payments Counter.
- There is a *separate queue* for New Cases and for the Old Cases on the OPD Counter.
- There is a separate queue for ladies on the OPD Counter.

Salient Observations

- Some patients finding excessive time taken at the counter.
- Excessive time taken for searching the old patient medical record.
- Absence of queue discipline.

Staffing

- The hospital has **Honorary Consultants, Senior and Junior Consultants** on *contractual* and full time basis who take care of the various OPD's.
- The management of the hospital on the basis of their speciality appoints all of them. Many of them have served the Apex Government Hospitals and are the best in their respective speciality.
- Nursing Staff take care of the OPD's and helps the doctors in performing their duties efficiently and effectively.

A Few Of The Selected OPD's Are Discussed Below In Detail

GENERAL MEDICINE OPD

The multidisciplinary hospital has a well-equipped General Medicine OPD.

Location and Accessibility

It is located on the *ground floor* of the main hospital complex and is located in the corridor leading to the central lobby of the hospital. It is easily accessible by:

- Staircase,
- Ramp and
- Lifts.

Physical Facilities

It is located on the **ground floor** of the main hospital complex and has the following:

- 2 Consultation rooms
- 1 Dressing room
- Store
- Waiting space with Seating arrangement

Instruments and Equipment

- Instruments for dressing, stitch removing, catheterization
- Dressing sets
- Sphygmomanometer (BP apparatus with appropriate cuffs of different sizes)
- Stethoscope
- Clinical Thermometer
- Torch
- Aspiration sets
- Endotracheal tube
- Oxygen mask
- Oxygen cylinder
- Nebulizer chamber
- Metered dose inhaler
- Nelson's inhaler
- Ambu bag
- Mouth gag
- Simple rubber catheter
- Foley's self retaining catheter
- Urosac bag
- Stomach tube
- Ryle's tube
- Insulin syringe
- Examination beds
- X-Ray View Box
- Revolving Stool

Staff

- 3 Senior Consultants
- 3 Junior Consultants
- 1 Senior Registrar
- 1 Junior Registrar
- 6 Nurses
- 4 OPD Attendants
- 2 Sanitary Attendants

Duty hours as per OPD Timings i.e.

9 A.M. - 1 P. M.

5 P. M. - 7 P. M.

Diseases in which Patients Reports To OPD

Patients report in this OPD for the following conditions:

- Fever
- Chest pain
- Dyspnoea
- Cough
- Hemoptysis
- Palpitations
- Syncope
- Diarrhoea
- Hepatitis
- Cirrhosis of liver
- Hypertension
- Malaria
- Typhoid
- Pneumonia
- Bronchieactasis
- COPD
- Lung abscess
- Rheumatic fever
- Ischemic heart disease
- Cardiac failure
- Shock

Functioning

Once the patient reaches the OPD reception, they are examined by the consultant according to their number in the queue. If the patients come with minor ailment then he/she may be dispensed with prescription. If the patient has come with some ailment, which needs some other intervention, then that is performed as per clinical need of the patient.

Patients are advised different investigations if needed.

The major investigations ordered are:

- Haemoglobin concentration
- TLC
- DLC
- ESR
- X-Ray
- Ultrasound

Average Number of Patients seen Per Day

50

Peak Hours

10 A.M. - 11 A.M.

Average Consultation Time Per Patient

10 minutes

Records Maintained

- OPD register
- Stock register of consumables
- Injection register

Salient Observations

- Approximate turn in the queue is not conveyed to the patients who come with prior appointment.
- Patients visiting to collect reports are given priority.

CARDIAC REHABILITATION OPD

The multidisciplinary hospital has a Cardiac Rehabilitation OPD.

Location and Accessibility

It is located at the *basement* of the main hospital complex and it is easily accessible to staff and cardiac patients by:

- Lift,
- Ramp and
- Staircase.

Staff

- 1 Consultant
- 1 Sister Incharge
- 2 Staff Nurses
- 1 OPD Attendant
- 1 Sanitary Attendant

Timings

Same as the OPD timings of the hospital.

Types of Patient's Reporting to the Cardiac Rehabilitation OPD

- OPD patient's of the hospital
- IPD patient's of the hospital
- Outside patient's

Functioning

Once the patient has suffered from any cardiac disease, he suffers from physical and psychological disorders and is not able to lead a normal productive life. It is for these patients that this OPD has been established. It helps to counsel the patient and helps to bring him back to normal routine of life. He/she is given psychological support, dieatry advice and is asked to gradually increase his/her physical activities. This helps the patient to get rehabilitated from the trauma that he/she has undergone due to his/her ailment.

NEUROSURGERY OPD

The hospital has well equipped Neurosurgery OPD where head injury patients come for treatment. The hospital has qualified Neurosurgeon who is MS and MCh in Neurosurgery and who looks after the patients attending the Neurosurgery OPD.

Location And Accessibility

It is located in the *basement* of the main hospital complex and is easily accessible to the staff and patients by:

- Ramp,
- Lift and
- Staircase.

Physical Facilities

Neurosurgery OPD is in the *basement* and it has the following:

- Consultant's Chamber
- Dressing room
- Minor OT (Minor Operation Theatre)
- Waiting space for patients is in the corridor

Instruments and Equipment

- X-Ray View Box
- Sphygmomanometer (BP apparatus with appropriate cuffs of different sizes)
- Stethoscope
- Clinical Thermometer
- Torch
- Revolving Stool

Staff and Duty Hours

- 1 Neurosurgeon 9 A.M. - 3 P.M.
- 1 Staff Nurse 9 A.M. - 5 P.M.
- 1 Senior Consultant
- 1 Junior Consultant
- 2 OPD Attendants
- 1 Sanitary Attendant

Types of Patients Attending Neurology OPD

- Outside Patients

Investigations Ordered in OPD

- EMG
- EEG

- CT Scan
- Ultrasound
- X-Ray

Sundays OPD is closed.

Average Number of Patient Seen in OPD Per Day

15 Patients

Average Waiting Time for Patients in OPD

15 Minutes

Functioning

Minor cases are treated in the Minor OT and major cases are being managed in the Major OT of the multidisciplinary hospital.

Records Maintained

- OPD register
- Appointment diary

SURGERY OPD

(Orthopaedic and General Surgery)

The multidisciplinary hospital has a well-equipped Surgery OPD where minor surgical procedures can be performed.

Location and Accessibility

It is located on the *ground floor* of the main hospital complex and it lies in the corridor leading to the central lobby of the hospital. It is easily accessible by:

- Staircase,
- Ramp and
- Lifts.

Physical Facilities

It is located on the **ground floor** of the main hospital complex and has the following:

- 3 Consultation rooms
- 1 Dressing room
- 1 Plaster room /Procedure room/Minor Operation Theatre (OT)

- Store
- Waiting space with Sofas

Instruments and Equipment

- Sphygmomanometer (BP apparatus with appropriate cuffs of different sizes)
- Stethoscope
- Clinical Thermometer
- Torch
- Instruments for dressing, stitch removing, catheterization
- Dressing sets
- Aspiration sets
- Operation Theatre light
- Examination beds
- Plaster Saws
- X-Ray View Box
- Revolving Stool

Staff

- 3 Senior Consultants
- 2 Junior Consultants
- 1 Senior Registrar
- 1 Junior Registrar
- 6 Nurses
- 2 Plaster Technicians
- 4 OPD Attendants
- 2 Sanitary Attendants

Duty hours as per OPD Timings.

Diseases in which Patients Reports to OPD

Patients report in this OPD for the following conditions:

- Fractures
- Dislocation of joints
- Appendicitis
- Cholecystitis

Functioning

Once the patient reaches the Surgery OPD reception, he/she is examined by the consultant according to his number in the queue. If the patients come with minor ailment he may be dispensed with prescription. If the patient has come with some ailment, which needs some minor surgical intervention then that, can be performed in the Minor OperationTheatre.

In the case of uncomplicated fracture the same can be put into the plaster cast in the OPD.

Patients are adviced different investigations if needed by the consultants.

Major investigations ordered are:

- Haemoglobin concentration
- TLC
- DLC
- ESR
- X-Ray
- Ultrasound

If the patient is suffering from some ailment, which needs some major surgical intervention such as acute appendicitis and complicated fractures then, the interventions are made in Major OT's of the hospital.

When the patients come for follow up or removal of plaster the same is managed in OPD.

Average Number of Patients seen Per Day

30

Peak Hours

10 A.M. - 11 A.M.

Average Consultation Time Per Patient

10 minutes

Records Maintained

- OPD register
- Stock register of consumables

Salient Observations

- Approximate turn in the queue is not conveyed to the patients who come with prior appointment.
- Patients visiting to collect reports are given priority.

PAEDIATRICS OPD

The multidisciplinary hospital has a well-equipped paediatric OPD.

Location and Accessibility

It is located on the *first floor* of the main hospital complex. It is easily accessible by:

- Staircase,
- Ramp and
- Lifts.

Physical Facilities

It is located on the **first floor** of the main hospital complex and has the following:

- 2 Consultation rooms
- 1 Dressing room
- Store
- Waiting space with Seating arrangement

Instruments and Equipment

- Detecto scale
- Spring balance
- Non-stretchable fibre-glass tape
- Sphygmomanometer (BP apparatus with appropriate cuffs of different sizes)
- Stethoscope
- Clinical Thermometer
- Torch
- Revolving Stool
- Instruments for dressing, stitch removing, catheterization
- Dressing sets
- Aspiration sets

- Endotracheal tube
- Oxygen mask
- Oxygen cylinder
- Nebulizer chamber
- Metered dose inhaler
- Nelson's inhaler
- Ambu bag
- Mouth gag
- Simple rubber catheter
- Foley's self retaining catheter
- Urosac bag
- Stomach tube
- Ryle's tube
- Insulin syringe
- Examination beds
- X-Ray View Box
- Hammer

Staff

- 2 Consultants
- 2 Junior Consultants
- 1 Senior Registrar
- 1 Junior Registrar
- 8 Nurses
- 4 OPD Attendants
- 4 Sanitary Attendants

Duty hours as per OPD Timings.

Diseases in which Patients Reports to OPD

Patients report in this OPD for the following conditions:

- Signs of Vitamin deficiency in children
- Signs of Malnutrition in children
- Cerebral Palsy
- Rickets
- Cretinism

- Tetanus
- Glycogen storage diseases
- Fever
- Chest pain
- Dyspnoea
- Cough
- Hemoptysis
- Palpitations
- Syncope
- Diarrhoea
- Hepatitis
- Malaria
- Typhoid
- Pneumonia
- Bronchitis
- Rheumatic fever
- Shock

Functioning

Once the paediatric patient reaches the OPD reception, they are examined by the consultant according to their number in the queue. If the patients come with minor ailment then he/she may be dispensed with prescription. If the patient has come with some ailment, which needs some other intervention, then that is performed as per clinical need of the patient.

Patients are advised different investigations if needed.

Major investigations ordered are:

- Haemoglobin concentration
- TLC
- DLC
- ESR
- X-Ray
- Ultrasound

Average Number of Patients seen Per Day

50

Peak Hours

10 A.M. - 11 A.M.

Average Consultation Time Per Patient

10 minutes

Records Maintained

- OPD register
- Stock register of consumables
- Injection register

Salient Observations

- Approximate turn in the queue is not conveyed to the patients who come with prior appointment.
- Patients visiting to collect reports are given priority.

DENTAL SURGERY OPD

The multidisciplinary hospital has well equipped Dental Surgery OPD with one consultant taking care of the patients coming to avail the services of this OPD.

Location and Accessibility

It is located on the *first floor* of the main hospital complex and is easily accessible by:

- Staircase and
- Lifts.

Physical Facilities

It has the following facilities:

- One consultation room which is interconnected with one examination cum procedure room.
- Seating arrangement for the patients is in the corridor.

Instruments and Equipment

- Dental chair for examination and performing procedures on patients.
- Dental X-Ray unit to take X-Ray of teeth and mandibles.
- Ultra-violet light
- Ultra-sonic scaller to remove the plaque from teeth.

- Steriliser for sterilizing the equipments.
- Pneumatic Drill compressor.
- Vapour sterilizer for sterilizing instruments.
- X-Ray View Box
- Instant X-Ray Film developer, which can develop 8 films simultaneously in 8 minutes.
- Sphygmomanometer (BP apparatus with appropriate cuffs of different sizes)
- Stethoscope
- Clinical Thermometer
- Torch
- Revolving Stool

Miscellaneous Articles in OPD

- Mirror
- Geyser
- Wash basin
- Telephone
- Comics related to teeth and how to brush and to protect the teeth
- Dental cupboard with necessary articles
- Drugs for dispensing to the poor patients reporting to the OPD

Staff

- One Chief Dental Surgeon (BDS, MDS)
- One Auxillary Nurse Midwife (ANM)

Timing

Duty hours are same as OPD timings.

Diseases for Which the Patients Report to OPD

- Dental Carries
- Fractured mandibles
- Bleeding Gums
- Plaque
- Cavities

Functioning

Once the patient has arrived at the reception of OPD of Dental Surgery, the patient is registered by the Auxillary Nurse Midwife (ANM) and then the Dental Surgeon examines the patients. The Dental Surgeon carries out the following investigations if needed on the patient:

- Dental X -Ray
- Orthopentogram
- X-Ray
- Blood Test
- Urine Examination

If the patient has minor ailment then the patient is dispensed with prescription, however, if the problem is major then the patient is operated upon in the Operation Theatre (OT). For all minor procedures such as scaling, extraction of tooth etc. can be done in examination cum procedure room, whereas major surgery such as fractured mandibles or maxilofacial surgery is carried out in OT under general anaesthesia.

Patients who are allergic to local anaesthesia are also operated upon in OT.

When patient undergoes major surgery then the patient is admitted as IPD patient on the beds allocated for this speciality.

Wednesday and Friday are fixed for OT's.

Whenever a patient has to be given Local Anaesthesia (LA) or General Anesthesia (GA) then consent forms are to be duly filled and signed by the patient.

Registers Maintained

- OPD register
- Stock register for Capital Items

Peak Hours

9.30 A.M. - 11 A.M.

Average Number of Patients Seen Per Day

12

ENT OPD

The hospital has a well-equipped ENT OPD, which runs on alternate days of the week, as there are operation days in between.

Location and Accessibility

It is located in the *basement* of the main hospital complex and is easily accessible by:

- Ramp,
- Staircase and
- Lifts.

Physical Facilities

It is located in the *basement* of the main hospital complex in front of the Neurology OPD

It has the following:

- 2 Consultation cum Procedure Rooms
- 1 Consultation room for Speech and Audiology
- 1 Special Room for Audiometry and Speech Therapy which is sound proof
- Seating arrangements for the patients is in the corridor.

Staff

- 1 Consultant
- 1 Junior Consultant
- 1 Speech Therapist and Audiologist
- 2 Staff Nurses

Instruments and Equipment

- Bulls Eye Lamp for examination of ear, nose, throat and is used for focusing light
- Head Mirror for examination.
- Laryngoscope and auroscope
- Examination Set which includes the following:
    - ✧ Tongue Depressor
    - ✧ Nasal Speculum
    - ✧ Laryngeal Mirror
    - ✧ Ear Speculum

- Autoscope
- ENT Speculum
- X-Ray View- Box
- Suction Machine for aspiration of fluids
- Sphygmomanometer (BP apparatus with appropriate cuffs of different sizes)
- Stethoscope
- Clinical Thermometer
- Torch
- Revolving Stool
- Tuning Fork

Audiometry room has:

- Audiometer
- Tympanometer

Diseases in which the Patients Report to this OPD

Patients report for Ear, Nose and Throat diseases such as:

- Sinusitis
- Nasal Polyps
- Tonsillitis
- Deviated Nasal Septum
- Discharge from Ears
- Foreign body in Ear, Nose and Throat

Functioning

Once the patients report to the department, he/she is examined by the consultant. If it is needed, the following investigations are ordered:

- Blood Tests
- Urine Examination
- X-Ray Paranasal Sinuses
- Audiometry
- Tympanometry

If the patients need audiometry and speech therapy then the patient is directed to the room in the OPD specially meant for this purpose.

The following procedures can be performed in the OPD:

- ENT Examination and minor procedures can be performed
- Audiometry and Tympanometry
- Speech Therapy
- Removal of foreign bodies from Ear, Nose and Throat
- If a person reports with foreign body in throat then the same is removed in Operation Theatre
- Indirect Laryngoscopy

If the patients need to be admitted then the patient is transferred to *Speciality Ward* where 10 beds are allocated for ENT Speciality.

Peaks Hours

10 A.M. - 11 A.M.

Average Number of Patients Seen/Day

30 Patients

Average Waiting Time

10 Minutes

Records Maintained

- OPD register
- Waiting patients register (for Operations)
- Audiometry register
- Tympanometry register
- Speech therapy register

Salient Observations

- Waiting Space is common with Eye and Neurology OPD
- Audiology and Speech Therapy Room are separated by glass window

NEUROLOGY OPD

The hospital has well equipped Neurology OPD where patients having diseases of Central Nervous System come for clinical treatment. People suffering from Paralysis, Epilepsy, Haemeplegia, Quadriplegia etc. come to avail the services of Neurology OPD.

The hospital has qualified Neurologist who is MD and DM in

Neurology and who looks after the patients attending the Neurology OPD of the multidisciplinary hospital.

Location And Accessibility

It is located in the *basement* of the main hospital complex and is easily accessible to the staff and patients by:

- Ramp,
- Lift and
- Staircase.

Physical Facilities

Neurology OPD is in the *basement* and is in front of Speech and Audiology Therapy OPD and it has the following:

- Consultant's Chamber cum EMG room
- EEG Room
- Shoe Removing Room
- Waiting space for patients is in the corridor

Instruments and Equipment

- X-Ray View Box
- EMG Apparatus
- EEG Apparatus
- Sphygmomanometer (BP apparatus with appropriate cuffs of different sizes)
- Stethoscope
- Clinical Thermometer
- Torch
- Revolving Stool
- Hammer
- Pins
- Cotton

Staff and Duty Hours

- 1 Neurologist 9 A.M. - 3 P.M.
- 2 Staff Nurses 9 A.M. - 5 P.M.
- 2 Ward boys
- 1 Sanitary Attendant

Types of Patients Attending Neurology OPD

- Hospital Patients
- Outside Patients

Investigations Carried Out in Neurology OPD

- EMG
- EEG

EMG:

- It is Electromyography.
- Consultant performs it.
- It takes around 2 hours to do EMG.
- It is done on prior appointment.
- In case of emergency it can be done without appointment.
- Average EMG done is 4 per day.
- Report of EMG is given at the same time to the patient.
- Done on Saturday and Wednesday.

EEG:

It is Electroencephalogram.

- Staff Nurse can perform it.
- It takes around 30 minutes to do EEG.
- It can be done at anytime without any prior appointment.
- Average EEG done is 4 per day.
- Report of EEG is given after 2 P.M. from OPD.
- IPD reports directly sent to the respective wards.

Precautions

Hairs of the patient should be washed and there should be no oil in it. If oil is there then the electrodes do not stick properly and false reading will be reported.

It is done daily except on Sundays, as OPD is closed.

Average Number of Patient Seen in OPD Per Day

25 Patients.

Average Waiting Time for Patients in OPD

15 Minutes

Records Maintained

- OPD register
- EMG register
- EEG register
- Appointment diary for EMG

EYE OPD

The multidisciplinary hospital has an Eye OPD, which is well equipped to carry out minor procedures in the OPD.

Location And Accessibility

It is located in the *basement* of the main hospital complex and is easily accessible by:

- Ramp,
- Staircase and
- Lifts.

Physical Facilities

It is located in the *basement* of the hospital complex and has the following facilities:

- Consultation Room
- Nurses cum Reception Room
- Procedure cum Laser Room
- Waiting Space in the corridor
- Minor Operation Theatre

Instruments and Equipment

- Ophthalmoscope
- Laser for the treatment of Retina.
- Laser for treatment of Lens.
- Fundus Camera to take different photographs of the eye.
- Carotometer for measuring eye pressure.
- Slit lamps for examination of eye.
- Faucimeter for measuring spectacle number etc.
- Binocular Indirect Ophthalmoscope for examining eye.
- Torch for examining eye.

- Snellens Chart to measure vision.
- Laser Therapy Machine.
- Sphygmomanometer (BP apparatus with appropriate cuffs of different sizes)
- Stethoscope
- Clinical Thermometer
- Torch
- Revolving Stool

Staff

- 2 Senior Consultants
- 1 Junior Consultant
- 2 Resident Doctors
- 2 Staff Nurses
- 4 OPD Attendants
- 2 Sanitary Attendants

Diseases in Which the Patient Reports to OPD

- Cataract
- Glaucoma
- Diseases of Cornea
- Diseases of Iris
- Diseases of Retina
- Retinitis Pigmentosa
- Congenital Toxoplasmosis
- Stagardt's Disease

Average Waiting Time

20 Minutes

Average Patients Seen Per Day

12 Patients

Functioning of the OPD

Once the patient suffering from any eye disorder reaches the Consultant, the patient is examined thoroughly. The doctor, if needed carries out the following procedures in the OPD on the patient:

- Tonometry
- Angiography of Eye
- Foreign body removal from Eye
- Syringing and Probing
- Chalazion Treatment
- Field Charting

If the patient reporting to OPD has some major problem such as an injured eye, excessive bleeding etc., then the Consultant transfers the patient to the Operation Theatre (OT) and carries out the major surgery in the major OT's of the hospital.

Investigations Normally Ordered

- Blood Pressure (BP)
- Blood Sugar
- Tonometry

Records Maintained in the OPD

- Operation register
- OPD register
- Laser register
- Fundus Photography register
- Consultation register

Salient Observations

- Patients have to wait for a long time if the patient being examined has to be examined thoroughly.
- Some patients have to wait for only 2-3 minutes while others have to wait for 15-20 minutes to get examined.
- Seating arrangement is not adequate.
- More space should be allocated as the rooms are congested and movement becomes problematic.

DIETARY OPD

The multidisciplinary hospital has a dietary department and provides dietary services to the patients and also has a dietary OPD. Two full time Dietician takes care of the dietary services of the hospital.

Location And Accessbility

The dietary OPD is located in the *ground floor* and is easily accessible to the staff and the patients.

Physical Facilities

- 1 Consultation Room
- Waiting area with seating arrangement
- Toilet

Instruments and Equipment

- Weight Machine
- Height Measuring Scale
- Telephone
- Sphygmomanometer (BP apparatus with appropriate cuffs of different sizes)
- Stethoscope
- Clinical Thermometer
- Torch
- Revolving Stool

TIMINGS

Morning OPD	9 A. M. – 1 P. M.
Evening OPD	5 P. M. – 7 P. M.

Sunday is off

Staff

- 2 Consultants (Dietician)
- 1 Sister Incharge
- 2 Staff Nurses
- 2 OPD Attendants
- 2 Sanitary Attendants

Qualifications of Dietician

Postgraduate in dietetics

Types of Patients Availing The Services of The Dietician

- OPD Patients of the hospital

- IPD Patients of the hospital
- Outside Patients
- Health conscious people of the society

Conditions in Which The Dietician Services Are Required

- Obesity
- Heart Diseases
- Diabetes
- Kidney disorders
- Stomach disorder such as Constipation and Diarrhoea

Charges

The patient has to pay fees at the OPD Counter as per terms and condition of the Consultants.

Functioning of the OPD

Once the patient has reported to the dietician, the dietician does the following:

- History of the patient is taken.
- Checking the weight of the patient.
- Measuring the height of the patient.
- Discuss patient's preferences.
- Discuss about any other associated disease or problem.
- If needed the following investigation are ordered:
  - ✧ Blood Examination
  - ✧ Urine Examination
  - ✧ Stool Examination

Once the consultant has become aware of the physiological and pathological condition of the patient, the diet is planned according to the individual needs of the patient.

If the patient is from IPD and cannot report to the OPD the dietician goes to the IPD to see the patient or calls the attendant of the patient. Only prescription is issued at the OPD.

Follow Up after 8 days.

Average Time for Consultation With One Patient

20 Minutes

Average Waiting Time

20 Minutes

Average Patients Per Month

60 Patients

Peak Hours of OPD

10 A. M. - 12 Noon

Problems

Since it is difficult to change the attitude of the person specially regarding his or her diet the consultant at times find that, on follow up the patient has not accepted the advice and has not followed the prescription. Under such circumstances the consultant has to become strict with the patient.

Salient Observations

- Quality Dietary services are available in the multidisciplinary hospital.

MISCELLANEOUS OBSERVATIONS

Privacy in OPD's

- Patients have reported that most of the time privacy was maintained for them.
- In Gynaecology OPD 3 to 4 patients are provided service side by side by the consultants.
- Patients attempt to peep in to the doctors chambers in Orthopaedic OPD thus affecting the privacy of the patient being examined.
- In selected OPD's before the patient leaves the chamber the other patient enters.

Service Time in OPD's

- As reported by the patients, on an average the time taken to provide service to patients visiting without prior appointment with the doctor was 10 minutes for Medicine OPD.
- As reported by the patients, on an average the time taken to provide service to patients visiting without prior appointment with the doctor was 10 minutes for Orthopaedic OPD.

- As reported by the patients, on an average the time taken to provide service to patients visiting without prior appointment with the doctor was 7 minutes for Gynaecology OPD.

Outpatients Opinion on Investigations Suggested by Consultants

- Most of the patients found suggested number of investigations reasonable.

Outpatients Opinion on Location Convenience of OPD's

- Most of the patients found the location convenience of respective Consultant Chamber as good.

Cleanliness in OPD's

- Most of the patients reported that cleanliness was maintained in OPD's.

Drinking Water Availability in OPD's

- Most of the patients reported that clean drinking water was available in OPD's.

Public Telephone Availability in OPD's

- Most of the patients reported that **Public Telephone Service** was conveniently available in OPD's.

Seating Arrangment in OPD's

- Most of the patients reported that seating arrangement in OPD's was good.

Toilet's Facilities in OPD's

- Most of the patients reported that Toilet facility arrangement in OPD's was good.

Ventilation in OPD's

- Most of the patients reported that good ventilation in OPD's existed.

Dustbin Facility in OPD's

- Most of the patients reported that good dustbin facility was there in OPD's.

Outpatient Opinion on the Behaviour of OPD Staff

- Most of the patients reported consultants behaviour helpful and empathetic.
- A few patients reported unhelpful behaviour of OPD attendants.
- Most of the patients reported security personnel posted at OPD's as helpful and empathetic.

Outpatient Opinion on the Service Charges

- Most of the patients reported service charges at OPD's as reasonable.
- Repeat patients feel service charges high because of recurrent visits to OPD.

Outpatient Opinion on the Recommendation of the Hospital

- Most of the patients are willing to recommend the hospital to their relatives and friends.

DISCUSSION

The multidisciplinary tertiary care hospital is being managed in a highly professional manner by competent and dedicated clinical, paramedical and managerial staff. It is rendering its services to all the sections of the society and has a goodwill in the community. The catchment area of the hospital extends to several adjoining states. The hospital is equipped with the latest health care technology and is centrally air-cooled and totally computerized. It is delivering preventive, promotive and curative services to the community. It is delivering high quality services to the patients reporting for treatment.

There are some areas where further improvement can be made within the available resources at the disposal of the management. This will further lead to an increase in the operational efficiency of the unit. Most of the patients assessed reception of the hospital to be good but there is scope for further improving it. Queue discipline is not being maintained at the registration counter. There is delay in searching the old patient's medical records that leads to patient spending more time at the enquiry and reception counter. Moreover, the records are being handed over to the patients to carry to the consultant's chambers. The time reported to avail consultancy services was similar as reported by the patients. At times they have to wait for about more then an hour yet they find it acceptable. Patients find waiting space to be a little less especially during peak hours. Patients prefer to avail the services of the hospital even if the service charges are a bit high. Patients have expressed their satisfaction about the drinking water, ventilation facilities, toilet, public telephone services etc. available in the hospital. A large number of patients are highly satisfied with the various facilities offered by the hospital and are willing to recommend it to their relatives and friends. The various OPD's are situated separately and are not near the main entrance of the hospital, which leads to inconvenience to the patients coming to avail of its services.

RECOMMENDATIONS

In order to make the health care services being offered by the multidisciplinary hospital more efficient and effective the following recommendations are being made:

1. Due attention should be paid to clear the rush at or near the entrance of the multidisciplinary hospital.
2. Enquiry & Reception Counter should be located facing the entrance of the multidisciplinary hospital and the sign board identifying the counters should be appropriately located so that it is clearly visible to the patients coming to avail of its services.
3. There should be a board at the reception displaying the names of various consultants offering their services to the patients along with their respective speciality and location of their chambers.
4. Queue discipline should be strictly adhered at the various service counters of the multidisciplinary hospital in order to avoid any patient dissatisfaction.
5. Registration forms should be simple and at least in two languages i.e. Regional and English.
6. Proper filing of old patients medical records should be done so as to avoid delays.
7. Out-Patient Folder should be carried by hospital staff to the consultants chamber and patient should not be made to carry it.

8. Various consultants providing their services to the patients should be available during the OPD hours so that patients have not to wait for them.
9. Lifts should be operated by trained staff.
10. Seating arrangement should be increased in the various OPD's.
11. Facilities like clean drinking water, separate toilets for male and female etc. have to further improve so as keep the patient satisfaction levels high.
12. Timings of OPD's should be studied in detail in order to note the arrival patterns of the patient's and adjustments should be made if needed.

CONCLUSION

The multidisciplinary hospital has a well-equipped and managed Out-Patient Department with a range of services. OPD is providing high quality services to the community. It is professionally managed by competent and dedicated clinical, paramedical, nursing, support and administrative staff. There is scope for further improvement in the quality of services being provided by OPD.

REFERENCES

1. Ahmad, R., Tabish, S. A., Qadiri, G. J. and Mustafa, A. *Profile Of Patients Visiting Outpatient Department Of A Large Teaching Hospital,* Journal of the Academy of Hospital Administration, Vol.13, No.2, July - December 2001.
2. Goel, S.L. and Kumar, R. *Hospital Core Services,* Deep & Deep Publications PVT. LTD., New Delhi, 2004.
3. Hardy, O.B. and Lammers, L.P. *Hospitals The Planning And Design Process,* An Aspen Publication, Aspen Publishers Inc., Maryland, 1986.
4. Health Facility Planning *Design Primer,* Vol. 4, Hosmac (India) Private Limited, Mumbai, 2000.
5. Kumar, A. *Encyclopaedia Of Hospital Administration And Development,* Vol. 2, Institute For Sustainable Development Lucknow & Anmol Publications PVT.LTD., New Delhi, 2000.
6. Sreenivas, T. and Prasad, G. *Patient Satisfaction A Comparative Study,* Journal of the Academy of Hospital Administration, Vol.15, No.2, July - December 2003.

3

Organization and Management of Out-Patient (OPD) Services in Hospitals

- ★ Overview
- ★ History
- ★ Terminology
- ★ Functions
- ★ Types of Out-Patient Services
- ★ Work Load
- ★ Indices for Measuring the Efficiency of Out-Patient (OPD) Services
- ★ Monitoring Quality of Out-Patient Services
- ★ Patient Flow in Out-Patient Department (OPD)
- ★ Physical Considerations
- ★ Equipments
- ★ Staffing
- ★ Organization of the Out-Patient Department (OPD)
- ★ Managerial Considerations in Out-Patient Department (OPD)
- ★ Conclusion
- ★ References

OVERVIEW

Hospitals evolution of supporting sick from normal to care of sick and now it is sophistication of providing *preventive*, *promotive*, *curative* and *rehabilitative* services is phenomenal. As the hospital has grown in stature, so has its important arm, out-patient department. Out-patient services are an integral part of hospital services. Over 30 crore outpatients in a year are treated in the out-patient department of hospitals. The activities of out-patient departments have made the hospital a real force in the community programme, for the prevention of diseases. Much of the investigations and diagnostic work that formerly necessitated admission to hospital wards can now be carried out in a well-equipped out-patient department (Sakharkar, B.M, 1999). Out-patient department services are corollary to in-patient services in the form of general out-patient department, day care, home-care and rehabilitative centres (Alden B Mills, 1969). Out-patient services have evolved in hospitals in line with patient's needs, demands and expectations from a limited service offering basic and minor clinical services to a highly evolved and organized service.

The primary function of a hospital is patient care. The patient is the ultimate consumer to the hospital. The effectiveness of the hospital relates to provision of good patient care as intended. Medical care has been centered on the patient in the hospital bed. The *organization* of the hospital, the clinical and administrative services, the nursing, dietary and pharmacy services, and teaching and medical research have been focused on the admitted patient. This will continue to be true, but due importance must now also be placed upon the ambulatory patient in need of medical care. The rising cost of hospital and relative shortage of hospital beds with respect to needs tend to force hospital management to keep the hospitalization of patients down to the minimum. Modern health care practice with the concept of *active and early ambulation* tends also to shorten the period of rest in bed and hospitalization after the critical period is over. These patients after discharge will need some form of post-hospital treatment and rehabilitation in order to ensure complete recovery. At present much of the investigational, diagnostic and the therapeutic work that formerly required admission to a hospital can now be carried out in a well-equipped out-patient department, with a saving of expense and avoidance of the disruption of family life that occurs due to hospitalization.

Out-patient services when functionally integrated with the in-patient services of the hospital lead to continuity of medical care.

It is very important for health care planners to know about the *catchment area* of the hospital so that cost-effective and cost containment techniques will be employed before hospital gets commissioned.

Out-Patient Department (OPD) is a very important department of the hospital, which is visited by a large section of community. OPD is the first point of contact between patients, their relatives and hospital and its staff. The medical care provided in the OPD and behaviour of the staff determines the image of hospital in the minds of the consumers. OPD is referred to as "**shops window of the hospital**".

The out-patient department, requires an organization with a definite procedure and efficient and effective management. OPD is a part of, and co-ordinate with the organization of the hospital as whole. In an efficiently managed OPD the stay of the patients can also be significantly reduced, and the cost of care to the patient, hospital and the government can be brought down.

HISTORY

According to Sir George Clark the Out-Patient Department (OPD) as we know today originated in mid seventeenth century when at Hotel Dieu in Paris, six physicians were detailed for regular sessions on Wednesday or Saturday *advising the poor* individually. This lead to introduction of the idea of the out-patient clinic. Modern day OPD began to emerge in 1850 in USA from the framework of dispensaries. The main function of the OPD was a source of charity diagnosis, care and medicaments. At present OPD is used for both charity and paying patients.

TERMINOLOGY

Ambulatory Care: Out-patient care or services

Appointment System: After the first visit, the patients are given the date and time for their next visit.

Block Appointment: Calling for a certain number of patients to be present at a given time.

Filter Clinics: Clinics managed by nonspecialist general duty doctors who relieve congestion on speciality clinics.

Individual Appointment: Calling for a certain patient to be present at a given time.

Out-patient: A person given diagnostic, therapeutic or preventive service through the hospital's facilities and who, at the time is not registered as an in-patient in the hospital.

Out-patients can be grouped under the following categories:

Emergency Out-patient: A person given emergency care as a result of sudden severe illness or an accident. The need of emergency care is determined clinically. There are conditions considered by the patient or his/her relatives as requiring emergency services; the perception of "emergency" by patients or their relatives may be different from that of physicians.

Referred Out-patient: A person referred to the out-patient department by a private practitioner or other physicians from one clinical speciality to the other, for specific diagnostic or treatment procedures or opinion, and who will (or should) return to the referring physician for further care and disposal.

General Out-patient: A person not referred by other physician, given diagnostic and/or therapeutic services on an out-patient basis, for other than an emergency condition, his or her continuing care and disposal being undertaken by the out-patient department. General out-patients are those who come to the out-patient department on their own with a variety of ailments and regard the hospital as some kind of dispensary. They form the bulk of the users of the out-patient department in government run hospitals. A sizeable proportion of them may come for minor ailments because for them the hospital represents the only available source of medical care.

Out-patient Visit: An out-patient visit is the visit of a person at the out-patient department to receive service. The visit may be:

- **New out-patient visit**: out-patient visit by a person for the first time, or
- **Repeat out-patient visit**: out-patient visit by a person subsequent to initial out-patient visit.

Satellite Clinic: Clinics being located away from the main hospital OPD, to serve defined concentrations of populations, but having links with the main hospital.

Service Time: Service time is the time taken by the clinician to diagnose a patient's illness and in instructing him or her, and includes taking history, examination, making case note and prescription writing and signing requisitions for special medicines or investigations.

Unit of Service: Unit of service is a measurable part of the volume of service rendered in diagnostic or therapeutic facilities of the hospital, expressed in terms of time and quantity.

FUNCTIONS

Out-Patient Department (OPD) is one of the departments of the hospital, which cares for the ambulatory patient, who come to the department for diagnosis, treatment and follow up. The functions of out-patient services are to provide *diagnostic, curative, preventive* and *rehabilitative* services on ambulatory basis to the people of the community. The main functions of out-patient services, as listed by a WHO committee are as under:

- Early diagnosis of disease, using the best possible modern medical techniques, including prophylactic examinations for the detection of undiagnosed diseases.
- The ambulatory and domicillary treatment of all cases, which can be treated at the clinic or at home.
- The admission or referral for admission, to the hospital of those patients who need it.
- Aftercare and medical rehabilitation, when necessary after discharge from hospital.
- The promotion of health of the individuals under their care by means of health education.
- The use of out-patient facilities for the training of medical and nursing students.
- The keeping of medical records and collection of data for epidemiological and social research and for periodic assessment of medical work.

For carrying out the above functions, *continuity of care* is very important. There should be an easy transition of the patient from ambulatory and domicillary care to hospital care and back to his original physician.

The specific preventive medicine activities, which can be carried out by the out-patient department are:

- Well baby clinics and obstetric consultation, including marriage counseling and Planned Parenthood.
- School health programmes specially if the hospital is serving

a closed community like the armed forces or a factory establishment.

- Control of communicable diseases by early reporting, helping public health authorities in diagnosis and treatment, and carrying out specific protection on a limited scale.
- Control of epidemics by setting aside wards/beds for isolation of affected cases.
- Early diagnosis and detection of tuberculosis, cancer, rheumatic heart disease, syphilis, diabetes and psychiatric cases.
- Health education and advice on nutrition and dietetics.
- Rehabilitation and prevention of handicaps and disabilities.

Out-patient department is a very important wing of the hospital which is visited by a large section of the community. This is the first place where the sick and their relations come in direct contact with the hospital and its staff. The care and attention provided to them goes a long way in building up the reputation of the hospital and the confidence of the people in it. It is here that the human relation skills of the hospital staff are taxed to the maximum. As such the *public relations function* of the OPD, is of utmost importance. The staff working there have to be specially selected and trained to be polite, courteous, cheerful, cooperative and efficient. They should know the difficulties and limitations of their hospital and try to explain politely to the patients the reasons for minor delays and discomforts, which are bound to arise, being inherent in the situation.

TYPES OF OUT-PATIENT SERVICES

Out-Patient Services could be of the following types:

- **Centralized Out-Patient Services**: Here all the out-patient care relating to all the medical specialities are provided in a compact area which includes all diagnostic and therapeutics facilities also being provided in the same area. Polyclinic in various hospitals is based on centralized concept of out-patient services.
- **Decentralized Out-Patient Services**: Here the out-patient care is provided in the respective departments. The same holds true for diagnostic and therapeutic services provided by the hospital. The speciality clinics are based on decentralized out-patient services concept.

The use of *centralized out-patient services* or *decentralized out-patient services* in a particular hospital depends on the size, variety and workload of the hospital. It is seen that generally larger the hospital more centralized the out-patient services are. It also leads to economy as well as higher patient satisfaction. The patient satisfaction is the real testimony to the efficiency of hospital management. Satisfaction or dissatisfaction refers to emotional response to the evaluation of service, consumption and experience (Sreenivas, T. and Prasad, G., 2003).

WORK LOAD

Current statistics indicate that per hospital bed, 1.5 to 3 patients attend the out-patient department of a hospital per day. A 300 beded hospital should hope to cater for 450 to 900 out-patients a day. The attendance tends to rise towards the higher side of the scale as the bed strength of the hospital increases, although the converse is not always the case (Sakharkar, B.M, 1999).

The number of patients visiting the out-patient department will depend upon the following:

- The location of the hospital.
- The population and their needs.
- The programme and resources.
- The season of the year.
- Traffic and transport facilities.

In view of the above, the number of out-patients expected is not necessarily related to the number of beds in the hospital. With greater emphasis on out-patient and domiciliary services, the range of work in the out-patient department is increasing. The extent of facilities, which would be provided in any hospital, would depend on the objective of the hospital and the size of the community served by it; the workload may have a direct correlation, with the extent of facilities in the form of services provided. For the purpose of planning, a rough estimate might be to expect an average maximum of 500 out-patients for each hospital bed during a year: about 40 per cent of these would be new and 60 per cent old patients (Mc Gibony, Jr.).

It is a common complaint everywhere that the out-patient departments are overcrowded and that patients have to waste a considerable part of their time in waiting at different places. A Work-study conducted by COPP brought out the following probable reasons for overcrowding:

(a) Wrong placing of certain departments such as injection room, casualty department, dispensary, etc.

(b) Restricted registration time.

(c) Absence of appointment system.

(d) Shortage of medical staff in clinics.

Hospital clinics function for about five to six hours a day - three to four hours in the morning and one or two hours in the afternoon. In its report the COPP pointed out that in some hospitals a doctor in charge of a clinic had to examine about 25 to 40 patients per hour. This is considered to he excessive as a doctor should not be expected to attend to more than about 10 patients (new and old) per hour.

But, due to shortage of medical personnel this number has to be exceeded but no doctor should be expected to attend to more than 20 patients, old and new, per hour. On this basis, the other connected facilities should be determined.

Projection of Outpatient Load for Selected Target Area

The demand of out-patient care is expressed on per capita per year basis. This may vary from 1 to 10 visits per person per year, including revisits.

Projection of out-patient demand in a given area depends on:

- Unmet needs of the community for general medical and surgical care.
- Potential of cases being referred by General Practitioners (this will have a bearing on the demand on speciality clinics rather than on general medical and surgical clinics).
- Alternative health care services available in the area.
- Reputation and goodwill of the hospital.

INDICES FOR MEASURING THE EFFICIENCY OF OUT-PATIENT (OPD) SERVICES

1. **The Average Out-Patient Admission** = A ÷ B

   A means the total number of out-patients during the year

B means the total number of out-patient admissions during the year

2. **Average Daily Out-Patient Admissions** = A ÷ B

   A means the total number of new out-patients admissions during the year

   B means the number of working days during the year

The index tells the average *work load* on OPD services (Kumar, A., 2000).

MONITORING QUALITY OF OUT-PATIENT SERVICES

Quality is defined as a process of matching or achieving the standards already laid down for various functions or services. It is a multi-aspect concept. It refers to the quality of the individual professional as well as co-operation of professionals with respect to the whole organization. The concept of quality in health care could be easily deduced from the concept of quality in a professional service firm. Health care service quality is giving patients what they want (patient quality) and what they need (professional quality), and doing so using the fewest resources, without error, delays and waste, and within higher-level regulations (management quality) (Ovretveit 1992). The quality of out-patient services need to be monitored and evaluated on an ongoing basis in order that areas requiring attention for improvement could be identified as well as outcome of efforts made for improvement of quality of patient care could be known. In order to achieve this purpose, data need to be *collected, compiled, collated, analyzed* and acted upon on a regular basis by a nodal officer in the hospital. The various data that is needed for such a process is as follows:

Volume

- Clinic/department-wise statistics of new and repeat visits on monthly and yearly basis.
- Percent changes in new and repeat visits over years in relation to availability of consultants and registration staff.
- Fluctuation in visits by days of the week (or month)-average, high, low.
- Determine adequacy and utilization of clinics from clinic schedules of preceding year to determine number of hours

the clinic was in session, multiply number of session hours by number of rooms to arrive at number of scheduled hours, and divide this by number of patients seen or average service time to evaluate adequacy of rooms. By estimating actual room hours scheduled and dividing by potential room hours, it is possible to determine the clinic efficiency rate.

Utilization and Vital Statistics

The number of people who account for total annual visit volume determines utilization (average number of visits per person per year). This figure should be broken down by vital statistics of the population (age and sex). Such information helps in deciding staffing, programme planning etc.

Visit Levels

New appointments - walk-in, scheduled, short follows-ups, annual physicals, well-baby, well-child check-up, immunization and complex treatments indicate whether utilization, staffing, distribution and amount of revenues need to be changed or kept at the same level.

Cost and Revenues

Cost effectiveness is a very important issue of different quality activities. Quality costing methods and an awareness of the economics of quality are both important in ensuring that future quality programmes are more successful, and are needed to fill a gap in many discussions about quality and in research into quality.

The cost of each service should be matched with revenues from respective service. As far as possible, each service should be self-supporting, else cross-subsidy system be developed. Direct patient care costs (costs directly incurred or attributable to the patient care) like salaries, cost of supplies consumed as well as indirect patient care costs (costs indirectly incurred or not directly attributable to the patient care) like free-care costs, cost of utilities e.g. water, electricity etc., should be calculated (Agarwal, A.K., 2001).

PATIENT FLOW IN OUT-PATIENT DEPARTMENT (OPD)

The patient flow on out-patient visits, usually progresses from enquiry and registration to waiting, then to examination rooms, and thereafter to investigation facilities, and lastly the pharmacy.

PHYSICAL CONSIDERATIONS

The Out-Patient Department (OPD) is an integral part of the hospital organization, collaborating clinically, administratively and physically with the In-Patient Department (IPD) in the diagnosis and treatment of disease. OPD of a hospital has functional and administrative links with the hospital of which it is a part. It may also also be linked with health centre, dispensaries, and satellite clinics dependent on it.

LOCATION AND PHYSICAL FACILITIES

OPD should be located adjacent or in close proximity to important *adjacent services* such as registration, medical records, admitting, emergency and social services of the hospital. The main problem of OPD's is over-crowding and inadequate resources to meet the large number and variety of people who visit the OPD daily. This has to be borne in mind while considering the siting, layout and physical facilities to be provided. OPD should be near the main road and close to the main hospital entrance with sufficient space to provide for parking of vehicles and to prevent noise and dust pollution. OPD should separate from in-patient wards and other departments of the hospital but connected with them. It is desirable to have OPD's of all specialities in the same complex so as to facilitate cross-references between various specialities. It is desirable to have OPD on *ground floor*. In cases of large teaching hospitals, which would mostly be multistoreyed, it may be more advantageous to have in-patient and out-patient departmental activities on *contiguous floors*.

Size

The size of the OPD depends upon the volume of attendance, the clinics provided and the extent of other facilities like laboratory, blood bank, health education programme, operating facilities, and an emergency department. It should be so laid out that it is capable of expansion.

According to Bureau of Indian Standards there are following space provisions for various zones: 2 square metres per bed for entrance zone, 10 square metres per bed for the ambulatory zone, and 6 square metres per bed for diagnostic zone out of a total of 60 square metres per bed for the total hospital area.

Siting

The following principles should be kept in view while siting an OPD.

- It should have a separate entrance and approach from the main road, with liberal space for parking of vehicles.
- It should be ensured that patient flow moves in one direction in a logical sequence and there is no undue back traffic.
- It should be able to share with the in-patient department all diagnostic facilities such as X-ray, biochemistry and pathology laboratory.
- It should be amenable to expansion without serious dislocation of clinical work.

Planning Considerations

(a) System
(b) Referral System
(c) Desirability
(d) Feasibility
(e) Availability

Demand Utilization Coverage Parameters

(a) Operational
(b) Quality of care
(c) Cost efficiency parameters
(d) Expectation and satisfaction

Layout

The various layouts that can be used are:

- The double loaded single corridor with rooms on each side of the corridor.
- The double corridor for entry from the opposite sides of the room.
- The triple corridor which provides two rooms of examination treatment rooms on each side of a staff corridor.

Planning

The physical facilities may be considered under four groups :

(a) Public areas (Entrance Zone)
(b) Clinical areas (Ambulatory Zone and Diagnostic Zone)
(c) Administrative areas
(d) Circulation areas

PUBLIC AREAS

- **Entrance**: It should be easily accessible and should have wide door, ramps and steps. Main entrance to the out-patients should have gentle sloping ramps, with rise not exceeding 5 per cent.
- **Traffic**: Traffic of patients, visitors and staff should be planned to reduce congestion and cross traffic, and to expedite flow in every possible way.
- **Reception and Enquiry**: This may simply be a desk or a counter located within the public area. A reception and enquiry counter in the OPD is essential at the entrance lobby from where patients seek information about the location of various clinics, registration procedures and other necessary information. It is located at a prominent place at the entrance of the department and also in close proximity to the emergency department of the hospital. The entrance lobby should be connected with public facilities and with a tea and snack bar. In order to isolate it from the noise that usually exists in such a place reception and enquiry can be enclosed in a *see-through cubicle*. A small room with glass panelled wall above a height of 1.10 metre and a swinging door or doors has been found to be very effective. It enables the patients to see the person manning the reception and enquiry from a distance as well as enabling this person to watch the activity all around. In the OPD of smaller hospitals, an open booth or counter will serve the purpose. It should be prominently signposted. It should be staffed during the working hours of OPD by an experienced and highly competent person. A person who has complete knowledge of the location of every single facility and activity of the OPD must be posted as *reception clerk*. He or she should be well mannered and cool-tempered with in-

finite patience to hear patients innumerable queries and answer them politely. Reception and enquiry should have good communication facilities through telephone and intercom sets with all clinics and other important areas in the OPD. An easily understandable guide map showing locations of all clinics and adjunct services units should be visibly displayed in this location.

- **Registration and Records Area**: All patients have to register at the out-patient registration counter. It should be located near the entrance. Railings should be provided for separate queues - new patients and old patients, and male and female patients. One counter 100 cm high and with work surface 60 cm wide and with file drawers is essential. One desk should be provided for 20 patients per hours. Two sq. metres per bed should be provided for out-patient medical records. Old patients will be sent directly to the concerned clinical departments. New patients will be directed to the registration desk where appropriate records will be completed before sending them to the clinical departments. The area and the number of registration desks will vary with the patient load, but one desk will be able to handle 12-30 patients per hour. Mc Gibony recommends that an index card for every patient old and new might be maintained in this area; if so, 5 to 25 file drawers for 10,000 to 50,000 cards, 3x5 (or 5x7) inches, will be required. Medical records of patients under treatment will be retained in the department responsible for their care. When treatment is concluded and the patient discharged by the department the medical record may be returned to the Registration and Record Area, to be retained there in the active files for a period of one year, after which they may be filed in the Inactive Records Storage Area. He recommends 2 to 3 sq. ft per bed for out-patient records. ***Types of Registration and Record System*** - The type of registration and record system that is practised has a bearing on the requirement of space and manpower. The various types are:
  - ✧ **Centralized registration and record system**: Here all out-patient visits are registered and record kept at one place. It has advantages of conserving manpower and space.
  - ✧ **Decentralized registration and record system**: Here each clinic like medical, surgical, paediatric, etc. has its own

registration counter and records room. The patient goes directly to the appropriate clinic for registration on being directed at the reception and enquiry. There will be no registration counters and no records room in the main reception and waiting hall.

- ✧ **Mixed system**: Here the patient's first visit is registered and out-patient card originated at the central registration, but subsequent visits are registered at the respective clinic where his or her; medical record is then kept. Only the new out-patients will use the registration counters, as repeat visits will directly be registered at the respective clinics.

- **Waiting Area**: This will be required adjacent to Registration and in each clinical department. The waiting area is provided at the scale of one sq ft per patient, with a minimum of 400 sq ft (COPP). The space provided in subsidiary waiting areas adjacent to various consultation, diagnostic and therapy areas is 8 sq ft per patient for 1/3 of the average daily attendance. The waiting area should display boards for information of the patients and public regarding names of doctors and nursing staff on duty during a clinic session. Arrangement for clean drinking water in the form of a water cooler and dispenser should be made, and space for one or more public telephone booth should be earmarked.
- **Public toilets** and washrooms, for males and females, at the scale of one for each 200 patients and visitors, must be provided. Adequate number of toilet facilities should be provided separately for males and females. A scale of 1 to 2 WCs for every 100 patients attending the OPD and at least one urinal for every 50 patients are recommended.
- **Snack bar**: This should be maintained in a sanitary manner. It should be located convenient to the main waiting area, but out of the flow of traffic. It should be maintained in a hygienic manner.
- **Wheelchair and Trolley Bay**: Some patients cannot walk, stretcher-trolleys or wheelchairs will be required to carry them through the department. Adequate parking space for the required number of stretcher-trolleys and wheelchairs should be catered for. Parking place should be provided at the very entrance to the OPD. Adjoining to the reception and enquiry room would be a good location. The issue and replenishment

of trolleys and wheelchairs can be organized under the overall control of the OPD administrator.

CLINICAL AREAS

OPD includes generally the following departments:

- Medical Department
- Surgical Department
- Ophthalmic Department
- ENT Department
- Maternity and Gynaecology Department
- Paediatric Department
- Psychiatry Department
- Dermatology and Venereology Department
- Orthopaedic Department
- Emergency Department
- Dental Department

Some hospitals may have superspeciality clinics like:

- Neurosurgery
- Neurology
- Cardiology
- Urology

Moreover, there are *ancillary facilities* such as, treatment sections, including minor operation theatre, injection, dressing and dispensary, auxiliary services of pathology, blood bank and X-Ray.

There is also a growing need for instituting health education programmes to educate the public in environmental hygiene and family planning etc.

The general requirements for the above clinics, as recommended by the COPP, are given below:

- **Waiting area**: In addition to the principal waiting area provided at the entrance, subsidiary waiting areas will be necessary close to the consultation and treatment rooms. It has been estimated that at the peak, the number of persons waiting at any one time in the area is not more than one-third of the total number of patients visiting the clinic in a day. Based on this, waiting area may be provided at the rate of 8 sq ft per patient for one-third of the maximum number of the patients attending the clinic in one session.

- **Consultation room**: The cubicle should provide accommodation for a doctor's chair and table, patient's stool, follower's seat, washbasin, examination couch and equipment for clinical examination of the patients. Considering the sizes of the furniture, equipment and the extent of clear space required, the size of the cubicle should be about 160 sq ft. Maximum space in reality given is 120 sq ft. Each department may have more than one clinic depending on the volume of attendance. On an average each clinic will be able to handle 100 cases per day. It is important to see that the privacy of consultation is assured and the flow of patients is smooth.
- **Special examination room**: Certain departments like Medical, Eye, ENT and Psychiatry will need a separate room for special examinations, depending upon the type of equipment being used in the OPD. See table 3.1.

Table 3.1: Showing Area of Separate Rooms for Special Examinations in Some Departments

S.No.	Department	Separate Room	Area (Sq. Ft.)
1	Medical	ECG	150
2	E.N.T.	Audiometric	120
3	Psychiatry	EEG	100
4	Eye	Refraction Room	160
		Perimetry Room	120
		Tonography Room	120
		Slit Lamp Room	120

- **Treatment/dressing room**: The size will vary from 120 sq ft to 160 sq ft depending on the size of the department and the type of work carried out.

Ancillary Facilities

- **Injection clinic**: This clinic is provided for all out-patients needing injections prescribed on out-patient basis by the doctors. Patients requiring injection treatment with antibiotics, vitamin and other drugs of the entire OPD attend the injection clinic. This requires a waiting area for about 10 to 20 patients at the rate of 6 to 8 sq ft per patient. This may vary depending upon the workload. Large hospitals will need two to four cubicles for treating men and women separately. The space requirement in large hospitals may be up to 400 sq ft. The injection clinic is staffed by a nurse. It should be of adequate size to accommodate an examination table for patient to lie down during injection, nurse's desk and chair, few chairs or stools for patients, a portable sterilizer, and a sink. Adequate storage space for injections and syringes in the form of a cupboard should be there. The clinic should be provided with an outlet from the central oxygen circuit and be equipped to deal with a case of *anaphylactic shock* if it occurs, with arrangements to call a medical officer within seconds should such a situation arise.

- **Pharmacy**: The hospital pharmacy or dispensary should be so located as to serve both in-patients and out-patients. The dispensary is generally the last department to be visited by the patients, who reach there in a tired state. It is, therefore important that the waiting–room is comfortable. The accommodation should be adequate to contain about 5% of the total clinical visits to the out-patient department in one session. The dispensing and compounding room will require multiple dispensing windows, compounding counters with sink, and drug storage cabinets and shelves. The area required should in no case be less than 250 square feet (sq. ft.) for even the smallest hospitals.
- **Dressing Room**: The dressing room will have space for a few chairs or stools and an examination table, dresser's desk and chair, a sink and adequate storage space for dressing materials. It will be staffed by a nurse or a nursing orderly specially trained in dressing wounds and ulcers. Some of the patients initially treated in the minor operation theatre needing subsequent dressings will also be attended here.
- **Minor Operating Theatre:** Ambulatory surgery is less complex than major procedure, which requires prolonged post-operative monitoring and hospital care. Quite a load of minor surgical conditions can be handled in the OPD itself if it has a facility to deal with such cases. This reduces the load on the main operation theatre suite of the hospital. Large, hospi-

tals may need more than one minor operation room with associated facilities. These, along with a number of recovery cubicles should enable the staff to treat more surgical patients as out-patients rather than in-patients. Because the out-patient department receives many patients needing intervention for abscesses, whitlows, ulcers, cuts and, foreign bodies, minor septic surgery is likely to form the bulk of the work of this operating theatre. The design of this theatre will not be as elaborate as the hospital's main operation theatre. Since the nature of operations also does not call for several assistants or bulky accessory equipment that is normally required in operation theatre, an area of 20 m^2 is considered sufficient. A recovery room should be provided additionally. This room would also be used as a plaster room for uncomplicated fracture cases.

Auxilliary Facilities

- **Laboratory**: The hospital laboratory should be so situated as to serve both in and out patients. However, a sample collecting station for urine, stool and blood specimens should be provided separately in the OPD. This would consist of two (male and female) wash rooms and toilets (150 sq ft) and a bleeding room (150-200 sq ft) with two or more examination tables. In large out-patient department it will be advantageous to have a side room attached to the collecting station for routine examination of blood, urine and stool The exact design and equipment must be decided in keeping with the programme and services to be rendered.
- **Radiology**: Like the laboratory and pharmacy, the X-Ray department of the hospital should be so located as to serve both in-patients and out-patients. Radiology is an essential part of investigations for out-patients in addition to the clinical laboratory. It is known that up to 50 per cent of new out-patient visits result in radiological investigations.
- **Blood Bank**: This should be conveniently located near the OPD to serve both out-patients and in-patients. The unit will include, a reception-cum waiting room, bleeding room, laboratory for grouping, recovery room and a room for storage of blood and ancillaries like washing and sterilization room, office room and toilet facilities.

- **Health Education**: Health education is one of the most important functions of any out-patient department. The out-patient department is the connecting link between the hospital and the community. It can be an important agent in the prevention of disease and promotion of public health. For these reasons, it is desirable to have space allotted in the out-patient department area for the purpose. It will serve as an office for the health educator, as a conference and lecture room, and for display of educational material. One or more individuals trained in special methods of health education will pay huge dividends by assisting the staff to promote better health among patients and the community served. The minimum desired area would be 150 sq ft (double this in larger hospitals) with a desk, a chair, conference chairs, black board, cork bulletin board, screen, projector and visual aid materials such as TV, Video player and health education cassettes.
- **Medical Social Service**: The purpose of the medical social service is to assist in meeting the problems of patients whose medical needs may be aggravated by social factors, and who need this assistance in order that clinical services are fully effective (Mc Gibony). For this reasons, a unit of the social service department of the hospital should be allocated space in the out-patient area. A suitable cubicle for each social worker/counselor to provide privacy should be there in the OPD. For a larger hospital with several social workers, an interview cubicle for each worker is necessary.
- **Screening Clinic**: This is specially required in a tertiary care and teaching hospital. The department of medicine is normally responsible for cursory examination of new patients to decide as to which department they should report for definitive examination and treatment. Space for this should be located convenient to the Registration - Reception area and should consist of one or more cubicles with examination table, and stool, a table and a chair. One to four such cubicles, each lOx12 ft., should be there. This reduces the workload on the speciality clinic and also increases the quality of care of speciality services. Such an area offers a potential for development of a General Practice Clinic (Mc Gibony) needed for a teaching institution. In such a programme there is definitive

examination, treatment and follow-up of selected individual and family cases.

- **Preventive and Social Medicine**: Along with medical care, education and research, a good hospital discharges an important responsibility in preventive aspects of community health care. Control of communicable diseases, sanitation, immunization, well baby and well adult clinics and instruction, nutrition, home care, public health, nursing, morbidity and mortality studies, records and reporting, mental health, occupational hazards, education and general attention to social and economic aspects of health are but a few of the important functions of a department of preventive and social medicine. Facilities for this focal point will vary with availability, interest and enthusiasm of personnel The minimum would be at least an office of size 150 sq ft.

ADMINISTRATIVE AREAS

- **Administrator's Office**: The out-patient department will require an administrator in large hospitals. In hospitals of 100 beds or more planning, organizing, supervising, evaluating, coordinating and improving out-patient services requires a full time staff member. A room of 150 sq ft. is required.
- **Business Office**: This is an extension of the main business office of the hospital and may be provided in large and active OPDs. This may be utilized for personnel actions, requisitions, making reports and so on.
- **House-Keeping**: Every floor should be provided with a janitor's closet for house-keeping and cleansing materials. The size of the room may be 40 sq ft.
- **Storage Facilities**
  - ✧ **General Store**: As a rule, general stores for the OPD will be handled in the general storage area of the hospital
  - ✧ **Drugs Store**: Pharmacy stores are kept in the hospital drug store at a central place.
  - ✧ **Linen Storage**: Each floor of the department will require a closet, with shelves, for storage of daily supplies of linen. An area of 20 sq ft is required.

CIRCULATION AREAS

Circulation areas include corridors, stairs and lifts etc. It occupies about 30% of the total building area, elevators should be easily accessible specially for cardiac and obstetric patients. Corridors should be at least 1.8 metre wide. Security post should be provided at strategic locations. STD/ISD telephone facility also should be made available.

The Table 3.2 summarizes the areas (square feet) required in hospitals of different bed strengths.

Table 3.2: Hospital Bed Complement and the Areas Required (Square Feet) (Mc Gibony)

Number of beds In Hospital	50	100	200	300	400	500
Public Areas	1025	2125	3000	3400	4300	4350
Clinical Areas	5655	7105	12205	14695	17525	20815
Administrative Areas	2260	2960	4020	5280	6200	7000
Circulation Areas*	3060	3810	5175	6625	7965	9835
Total Net Area	12000	16000	24400	30000	36000	42000
Wall and Partition Areas (10%)	1200	1600	2000	3000	3600	4200
Gross Area for Total Building	13200	17600	26400	33000	39600	46200

* Circulation areas include corridors, stairs, lifts etc. In an averge building, such space will amount to about 30% of the total building area.

EQUIPMENTS

Equipments as required to the speciality examination should be made available in the concerned room. Sufficient numbers of wheelchairs and stretchers in a suitable, accessible location should be there. Each consultation-cum-examination room should have:

- A work table
- Physicians desk
- Wall mounted cabinets
- X-Ray View Box

- Revolving stools
- Chairs
- Examination couch
- Wash basin
- Instrument trolley

It is mandatory that all OPDs should have equipments for resuscitation of patient collapsing suddenly.

STAFFING

Staffing levels for the out-patient services should be dependent on analysis of the objectives of the department and on the volume of the workload in each of its functional areas.

The out-patient department will require an administrator in large hospitals for planning, organizing, supervising, evaluating, coordinating and improving out-patient services.

Receptionists, who make the first contact with the staff, are important members of out-patient staff.

There should be no separation of medical staff into in-patient and out-patient staff so as to ensure continuity of high quality care. The nursing staff consisting of qualified, competent and registered nurses, ANMs and nursing or hospital aids in sufficient number should be provided in the OPD. Ancillary staff in OPD e.g. X-ray, Laboratory, EEG and ECG technicians also are needed. Clerical staff is required in OPDs. The clerical staff carries out registration, patient's billing, cashiering, secretarial and medical record functions. In teaching hospitals, senior consultants have interns and senior and junior residents assisting them in delivering professional care to patients. Some hospitals use volunteers in a variety of activities in the out-patient services.

ORGANIZATION OF THE OUT-PATIENT DEPARTMENT (OPD)

Out-patient department is defined as a part of the hospital with allotted physical facilities and medical and other staff in sufficient numbers, with regularly scheduled hours, to provide care for patients who are not registered as in-patients (Sakharkar, B.M, 1999).

Policies and Procedures

Keeping in view the interdependence of the staff, facilities and services of the hospital with that of the out-patient department it is essential that policies and procedures for each aspect of its functioning should be laid down in writing and be documented in a retrievable format. Policies are guidelines for action in all situations in general. Procedures aim at putting the policies into practice and in adapting the facilities to the operational need, and are thus standardized methods of work. To run the out-patient department efficiently and efficiently, these should cover both managerial and technical aspects of the out-patient services.

The basic policy in the out-patient department should be to achieve continuity of high quality patient care with modern health care techniques and methods in order to have total patient satisfaction at all times with the willing co-operation of all the health care staff working in the out-patient department as well as in-patient departments.

Procedures

There should be a manual of the procedures to be followed by all health care staff working in the out-patient services. Each health care personnel should be trained and retrained in carrying out all or any procedure related to their work area. The various procedures carried out in the out-patient department should be carefully recorded and documented in a retrievable format so that the patient can be benefited in future as well as outcome of treatment could be scientifically evaluated.

It is good to implement appointment system to spread out the reporting time of patients. This can be either **individual** or **block appointments**. The block appointment system calls for a certain number of patients to be present at a given time so as to provide a sufficient pool of patients; thus the physician will at no time find himself idle and it limits the pool to the capacity of the waiting room. The consultant must keep a few *appointments vacant* to serve for serious patients who may have to be attended out of turn.

Information, graphics and signage system, name boards, pictorial representation of services provided, direction signs, colour coding of different service areas facilitate in easy understanding of hospital procedures and routines by the patients.

Functional Relationship

Having discussed earlier the extent of facilities and their space requirements, the next step is to consider their functional relationship. In the out-patient department the care of the ambulatory patient is the main consideration. In order to achieve maximum efficiency, a highly *systematized routine* is necessary, and there must be perfect coordination with the in-patient departments and the diagnostic facilities of the hospital The main considerations are:

- Within the OPD, the physical facilities should be placed ensuring smooth flow of operation, and easy and quick intercommunication.
- Services common to both the in-patient and out-patient departments should be readily and easily accessible from the OPD and should not involve undue effort in movement (Radiology, Laboratory, Blood Bank).
- Compilation of a programme of clinics on a weekly or other suitable basis.
- Provision of sufficient doctors and nurses and other necessary staff, with arrangements for holidays, sick leave and other absences.
- Provision of adequate auxiliary department and facilities on a scale which permits efficient handling of the load.
- Installation and review of an appointment system based on the doctors' rates of working.
- Review of the detailed arrangements from the point of view of amenity for patients.

MANAGERIAL CONSIDERATIONS IN OUT-PATIENT DEPARTMENT (OPD)

Public Relations

Public relations can be defined as the image of a hospital by the users and their peer groups (Sakharkar, B.M.1999).

Due to a growing appreciation of human values couples with improved socio-economic conditions, the community's expectations from hospitals have undergone a great change.

OPD is their first point of contact with the hospital for many members of the community. Therefore, it should be something of a showpiece making evident from the first the warmth and humanity of the hospital, its respect for the patient and his dignity, its provision of the proper setting for good clinical care, and its good management. Many of these things the patient can and will judge for himself and they may influence unduly his future opinions about the hospital. All efforts must be so directed that the impression the patient gets in the OPD is a favourable one.

Overcrowding and Long Waiting Time

It is commonly seen that many hospitals face the problem of overcrowding and long waiting time. Due to various reasons, patient after initial waiting for registration waits for consultations, diagnostics, treatment or even for collection of medicines at pharmacy.

Adequate attention by all hospital management must be given to solve this problem. A simple random study of waiting patterns since the arrival of patients through his final disposal and reasons thereof must be carried out and bottlenecks removed. The queuing theory can be applied to resolve the problem. Queuing and waiting line problems can be managed by the following methods:

- Appointment System
- Satellite Clinics
- Filter Clinics
- Starting OPD in Time and Prolonging OPD Timings

OPD Timings

The OPD timings should be decided to suit the local and hospital needs. General OPDs with basic specialities are usually conducted six days in a week may be from 0800 hr to 1300 hr or so. All registered patients must be seen irrespective of the timings fixed for OPDs. Timings for ancilliary/supportive facilities must be kept at least one hour after the OPD timings so that no patient who has been seen in the OPD is denied the treatment, investigation or drugs. It also must be ensured by the administrator that the timings for OPD are strictly followed. Increase in registration time, adequate number of doctors, separate queue for new or old cases may help in reducing waiting time in registration.

Screening clinics help in disposal of patients with minor illnesses thus leading to less crowding and waiting time in speciality clinics. Special clinics at different timings, specially during afternoon hours, e.g.,well-baby clinic, diabetes clinic, leprosy/TB, follow up, super speciality clinics etc. also prevent overcrowding in OPDs. Increasing the duration of OPD services or operating evening OPD services can also prevent overcrowding. Synchronizing functioning of ancillary facilities with OPD work load such that the laboratory, radiology and pharmacy are open and adequately staffed during peak hours when patients referred from the OPD arrive for these services is a managerial technique to increase patient satisfaction. These departments should remain open for a longer duration as compared to OPD.

The patient's medical records of indoor and outdoor services, investigations and treatment should be available in an easily retrievable form at each visit by the patient.

Management Structure

This may vary among hospitals. In larger hospitals, the Medical Director or the Medical Superintendent may be directly incharge of out-patient department. He / she may have assistants in various units such as clinics, outpatient surgery etc. reporting to him. In smaller hospitals, there may be a co-ordinator to co-ordinate the work of various units of the department reporting to the Medical Director or the Medical Superintendent. In some hospitals the Deputy Medical Superintendent may be made responsible for OPD services and he/she reports to the Medical Superintendent.

The nursing side of the OPD should be the responsibility of a well-qualified and experienced nurse incharge whose primary function should be to see that the work, in the various clinics proceeds smoothly and efficiently. She will direct the activities of the nurses and ancillary personnel who work permanently in the OPD.

CONCLUSION

Good out-patient services constitute one of the most important elements of a good hospital. Planning and provision of sufficient number of hospital beds, although desirable, is economically impossible. We have to, therefore, depend more on out-patient services to meet the growing health needs of the people through health education prevention, early diagnosis, case finding, better diagnostic and therapeutic procedures, and rehabilitation and follow-up, all of which are a challenge to sound planning and good administration of the out-patient department (Mc Gibony).

The timings of OPD should be decided to suit the local and hospital needs. It is good to implement *appointment system* to spread out the reporting time of patients. The basic policy in the OPD should be to achieve continuity of high quality patient care with modern health care techniques and methods in order to have total patient satisfaction at all times with the willing co-operation of all the health care staff working in the out-patient department as well as in-patient departments.

A good out-patient department is far more than merely buildings and equipment. These are facilities which make it possible, or easier, to discharge the responsibility, i.e. the care of sick people by health professionals. Such care can be furnished to the satisfaction of the patient, the public the medical staff and others concerned, only if administrative organization and execution is *alert, dynamic* and *understanding.*

The functions of out-patient services have gradually widened over the years. Out-patient services provide for the community a major source of specialist diagnostic medical opinion where the knowledge skills and resources of the specialist are backed up by the resources of the hospital. It includes not only the physical resources but also the presence of a wide range of other specialists that facilitates early *referral* when necessary and of supportive paramedical staff of the allied health professions. OPD treats on ambulatory and domiciliary basis all cases, which can be treated in the Out-Patient Department. It refers patients for admission to the hospital of those who need it. OPD carries out after care and medical rehabilitation, when necessary, after discharge from hospital. It promotes health of the individuals under care by means of health education. OPD trains medical students, house physicians, house surgeons and other professional medical staff such as nurses and technicians with valuable and diversified clinical experiences. Efficient, organized and professionally managed OPD has a role to compile, collate and analyze records of patients using out-patient services for epidemiological, social, clinical research and for periodic assessment of clinical outcomes. OPD carry out preventive and promotive services through provision of:

- Immunization
- Screening
- Antenatal Clinic
- Well-baby Clinic

- Counselling
- Family Welfare Clinics

REFERENCES

1. Agarwal, A.K *Clinical Services-1*, Indira Gandhi National Open University, School of Health Sciences, New Delhi, 2001.
2. Alden B Mills *Functional Planning Of General Hospitals*, American Association of Hospital Consultants, 1969.
3. Chester, T.E *Prevention and Health Care Costs*, World Hospitals, 22(1): 1986.
4. Cox, A. and Groves, P. *Hospitals and HealthCare Facilities – A Design and Development Guide*, Butterworth and Co. (Publishers) Ltd., 1990.
5. Davies, R.L. and MaCaulay H..M.C. *Outpatient Services in Hospital Planning and Administration*, WHO, Geneva, 1966.
6. Grant, Colin *Outpatient Services in Hospital Management*, Churchill Livingstone, Edinburgh, 1973.
7. Kteczowski, B. M., Piboulaeu, R.: *Approaches* to *Planning and Design of Health Care Facilities in Developing Areas* WHO, Geneva, I: 1977.
8. Kumar, A. *Encyclopaedia Of Hospital Administration And Development*, Vol.2, Institute For Sustainable Development Lucknow & Anmol Publications PVT. LTD., New Delhi, 2000.
9. Kunders, G.D., Gopinath Sand Katakam A. *Outpatient Services in Hospitals Planning, Design and Management*, Tata McGraw Hill Publishing Co. Ltd., New Delhi, 1999.
10. MAC Eachern, MT *Hospital Administration and Management*.
11. Mc Gibony, Jr. *Hospital Out-Patient Services-A Guide to Planning*.
12. Ovretveit, J. *Health Service Quality*, Blackwell Scientific Press, Oxford, 1992.
13. Ramaswamy, M. A., Murali, N. S. and Rao, K. V. *International Conference on Hospitals and Primary Health Care*, New Delhi, 1985.
14. *Reaction of Patients towards Evening OPD Services in Delhi Hospitals*, Hospital Administration, 14 (13) :1977.
15. Report of Hospital Review Committee, Delhi Hospitals, New Delhi, 1968.
16. Report on General Hospitals, Committee on Plans and Projects, New Delhi, 1964.
17. Role of Hospitals in Ambulatory and Domicillary Medical Care, WHO, Fecher Rep. Ser.,176, 1959.
18. Ross, H. R.: *Customer Service in a Hospital Outpatient Department*, Hospital and Health Services Review, 81(6): 1985.

19. Sakharkar, B.M. *Principles of Hospital Administration and Planning,* Jaypee Brothers Medical Publishers (P) Ltd., New Delhi 1999.
20. Shanon, K. *Outpatient Surgery. Hospitals* 59 (10) : 1985.
21. Sreenivas, T. and Prasad, G. *Patient Satisfaction A Comparative Study,* Journal of the Academy Of Hospital Administration, Vol.15, No.2, July - December 2003
22. Vogal, A. *Approaches* to *Planning and Design of Health-Care Facilities in Developing Areas,* WHO Geneva, II: 1979.
23. World Health Organisation *Role of Hospitals in Ambulatory Care and Domiciliary Medical Care,* WHO Technical Report Series 176, Geneva, 1957.

4

Research for Assessment of Out-Patient (OPD) Services of Hospitals

- ★ Overview
- ★ Meaning of Research
- ★ Objectives of Research
- ★ Motives for Doing Research
- ★ Types of Research
- ★ Significance of Research
- ★ Scientific Methods
- ★ Research Methodology
- ★ Research Process
- ★ Research Design
- ★ Sample Size
- ★ Queue
- ★ Materials and Methods for Assessment of Out-Patient Department (OPD) Services in Hospitals
- ★ Action Plan
- ★ A Research Plan for Studying the Operational Efficiency of OPDs in a Hospital
- ★ Checklist for a Visit to OPD Services
- ★ Points to remember while carrying out study of any live problems in OPD
- ★ Conclusion
- ★ References

OVERVIEW

Out-Patient Department (OPD) is the part of hospital with physical, medical and other facilities to provide care to patients who are not registered as in-patients. It includes Emergency OPD, General OPD and Referral or Speciality OPD. OPD is the first point of contact with patient. It is the stepping stone for health promotion and disease prevention. It acts as a filter, thus reducing the number of admissions into the hospital. The rising cost of hospitalization has enhanced the need to keep hospitalization to the minimum and thus enhances the importance of OPD services. It is an inseparable link in the hierarchical chain of progressive health care. A good OPD service reduces morbidity and mortality rates. Assessment of OPD services of a hospital is very important and it should be carried out by professionals trained in hospital and health care management in a scientific way so as to continuously improve the system of delivering OPD health care services to the community. A continuous improvement in quality of health care delivered by OPD will lead to a positive image of the hospital in the minds of consumers.

MEANING OF RESEARCH

Research can be defined as a scientific and systematic search for pertinent information on a specific topic. According to the Advanced Learner's Dictionary (1952) of current English, Research is "a careful investigation or inquiry specially through search for new facts in any branch of knowledge".

According to Redman and Mory, Research is "a systematized effort to gain new knowledge".

Research comprises of:

- Defining and redefining problems
- Formulating hypothesis or suggested solutions
- Collecting, organizing and evaluating data
- Making deductions
- Reaching conclusions
- Testing the conclusions to determine whether they fit the formulated hypothesis (Kothari, 1990)

There are various components of a research problem *viz.*:

- There must be an individual or group, which has some difficulty or the problem.

- There must be some objectives to be attained at.
- There must be alternative means for obtaining the objective(s) on wishes to attain.
- There must remain some doubt in the mind of the researcher with regard to the selection of alternatives.
- There must be some environment(s) to which the difficulty pertains (Ackoff, 1961).

OBJECTIVES OF RESEARCH

The main aim of research is to discover answers to questions through the application of scientific procedures. Research objectives fall in to the following groups:

- To gain familiarity with phenomenon or to achieve new insights into it (*exploratory* or *formulative* research studies).
- To portray accurately the characteristic of a particular individual, situation or a group (*descriptive* research studies).
- To determine the frequency with which something occurs or with which it is associated with something else (*diagnostic* research studies).
- To test a hypothesis of a causal relationship between variable (*hypothesis-testing* research studies).

MOTIVES FOR DOING RESEARCH

The main motives for doing research may be either one or more of the following:

- Desire to get a research degree along with its consequential benefits.
- Desire to face the challenge in solving the unsolved problems.
- Desire to get intellectual joy of doing some creative work.
- Desire to be of service to society.
- Desire to get respectability.

TYPES OF RESEARCH

The basic types of research are as follows:

- Descriptive vs. Analytical

- Applied vs. Fundamental
- Quantitative vs. Qualitative
- Conceptual vs. Empirical
- One-time research or Longitudinal research
- Field-setting research
- Clinical or Diagnostic research
- Historical research

SIGNIFICANCE OF RESEARCH

Research develops scientific and inductive thinking and it promotes the development of logical habits of thinking and organization.

SCIENTIFIC METHODS

There are two general traits that characterize a scientific method *viz.*:

- **Validity** – It is the characteristic used to describe research that measures what it claims to measure.
- **Reliability** – It is the characteristic of a research methodology that allows it to be repeated again and again by any researcher – always with the same results (Harper W. Boyd, Jr., Westfall, R. and Stasch, Stanley F, 1996)

RESEARCH METHODOLOGY

It is a way to systematically solve the research problem. It may be understood as a science of studying how research is done scientifically [Sinha and Chattopadhyay, 2003(a)].

RESEARCH PROCESS

The following provides a useful procedural guideline regarding the research process:

- Formulating the research problem
- Extensive literature survey
- Developing the hypothesis
- Preparing the research design

- Determining the sample design
  - ✧ Deliberate sampling
  - ✧ Simple random sampling
  - ✧ Systematic sampling
  - ✧ Stratified sampling
  - ✧ Quota sampling
  - ✧ Cluster sampling and area sampling
  - ✧ Multi-stage sampling
  - ✧ Sequential sampling
- Collecting the data
- Execution on the project
- Analysis of the data
- Hypothesis testing
- Generalizations and interpretations
- Preparation of the report or presentation of the results i. e. formal write up of conclusions reached

RESEARCH DESIGN

A research design is the arrangement of conditions for collection and analysis of data in a manner that aims to combine relevance to the research purpose with economy in procedure (Selltiz, 1962).

SAMPLE SIZE

The size of the sample depends on the following factors:

- Homogenicity and heterogenicity in the population
- Information about the population characteristic
- Sampling procedure
- Number of categories required for the analysis
- Spatial distribution of the population
- Precision of sample estimates (bigger the sample, greater is the precision) [Sinha and Chattopadhyay, 2003(b)]

QUEUE

A flow of customers from infinite/finite population towards the service facility forms a queue (waiting line) on account of lack of capability to serve them all at a time. The queues may be of persons waiting at a doctor's clinic or the railway booking office. Queues (waiting lines) stands for a number of customers waiting to be serviced (Swarup, K, Gupta, P.K. and Mohan, M., 1997)

MATERIALS AND METHODS FOR ASSESSMENT OF OUT-PATIENT DEPARTMENT (OPD) SERVICES IN HOSPITALS

The various tools and techniques, which can be used for assessment of OPD services of a hospital, are:

Visit to OPD: Principles of direct observation of OPD is to check the *accessibility*, *visibility*, *convenience* and *expandability* of the OPD. These four principles will help to assess the general planning of OPD e.g. the size, site, assessment of functional zones, etc. This would further help to get a view of the OPD process e.g.

- the waiting time,
- convenience,
- accessibility of services,
- the flow of patients.

Operational Research Techniques: By using operational research techniques one can quantify the services required for the given OPD and derive the solutions to the problems mathematically. The various operational research techniques, which can be used, are:

- Activity study/Work study
- Holding and lifting capacity
- Oueueing theory
- SWOT analysis

Review of the various policies and procedures: This will help to qualify and quantify the lacunae in physical facilities, equipment and stores, and activities found by the above methods.

Interview: Patients interview with the help of a questionnaire will go a long way in improving public relations both internal and external because a hospital is for its patients and patient satisfaction is the key to the services it provides.

ACTION PLAN

After reviewing the various materials and methods to assess the quality of service provided, one should concentrate on the exact plan of action. This implies, how the study should progress, the various details to be observed, analysis of results of various operational research techniques applied, reporting the results of questionnaire and interview which, one has developed.

These will help in qualifying and quantifying the problems and design alternate solution and select the best course of action amongst them.

Direct Observation

By direct observation it is meant that one should basically observe the structural and process criteria in OPD.

- See whether the location of OPD is easily visible to public, accessible and conveniently placed for the patient. This is a, subjective observation.
- See the adequacy of the size of OPD in context to the patient load and the extent of other facilities provided. McGibony has estimated a OPD load of two patients/bed/day.
- See the OPD site in relation to its need for:
  - ✧ Separate entrance without cris-crossing the in-patient services.
  - ✧ Sharing of investigation facilities with in-patients.
  - ✧ Unidirectional flow of patients.
  - ✧ Liberal parking space.
  - ✧ Space for future expansion.
- Assess whether the planning principle of "Design follows Function" holds good or not, i.e. whether the OPD has been divided into various functional zones or not.
- Public area should have:
  - ✧ Reception and Enquiry
  - ✧ 5% rise for ramp
  - ✧ An area for record keeping. Ideal is 5-25 file draw per 10-50,000 cards of 5" x 7" size.
  - ✧ An area for registration. McGibony recommended one registration desk for 12-30 patients per hour.

    - Waiting area: The main waiting area of OPD should be 1 sq.ft/patient with a minimum of 400 sq.ft.
    - 1 WC/100 patients and 1 toilet/50 patients.
- Clinical area should have:
    - Subsidiary waiting area i.e. waiting area in front of doctor's consultation room. It is estimated to have 8 sq.ft/patient for 1/3rd attendance in subsidiary waiting area.
    - Consultation room separate for each doctor with a screened area for examination which may be shared by two doctors. A consultation room should be at least 160 sq.ft.
    - Treating and dressing room for each speciality of 120-160 sq.ft.
    - Ancillary facility includes injection room and pharmacy.
    - Injection clinic should accommodate 10-20 patients at one time with a space requirement of 6-8 sq.ft per patient.
    - Auxiliary facility includes Laboratory, Radio-diagnosis, Blood Bank, Screening clinic and room for Medical Social Service Officer. Each of these area should constitute 150-200 sq.ft.
- Administrative area includes: It should be approximately 150 sq.ft.
    - Business Office
    - Housekeeping Service
    - Storage area for materials

McGibony has recommended that of the total area of OPD:

- Public area should constitute 10-15% of area
- Clinical area should constitute 40% of area
- Administrative area should constitute 15% of area
- Circulation area should constitute 25-30% of area
- Wall and partition area should constitute 10% of area

Evaluation of Process

The procedures and activities in the OPD can be evaluated by analyzing the various utilization pattern, flow of activity and use of operational research techniques.

Flow Concept: The flow concept defines the patient load in the various areas of OPD. This would help one to extend his services accordingly. It has been estimated that out of the patients coming for primary care in OPD:

- 20-40% attend injection room
- 5-15% attend the dressing room
- 5-10% attend the pharmacy/dispensary
- 5-10% go for the pathological investigations
- 2-5 % attend the minor theatre.

Holding capacity: Holding capacity is the adequacy of space to hold the patients in waiting areas. All OPDs with more than 2 floors should have lifts with adequate space.

Activity Sampling: Assess the utilization pattern of man and material in relation to workload by conducting an Activity Sampling. Activities of each category of personnel has to be defined and the time spent in each work has to be estimated. This is otherwise called as work study. This would also help in assessing the cost effectiveness of labour in OPD.

Material utilization has to be assessed vis-a-vis the workload, to analyze any wastage therein.

SWOT Analysis: The analysis of the Strength, Weakness, Opportunities and Threats of a hospital is a must before analyzing the services in its OPD. This would help in reviewing the policies and procedures of the service provided and seek necessary solution.

Queueing Theory: This is an operational research technique to quantify the waiting time of patients in each speciality and suggest alternate solution to reduce the queue and waiting time. The queueing theory has been developed in the attempt to answer the behaviour of queue, average waiting time and average time spent in the system. To study the queue one has to collect data of pattern of arrival of clientele, interval between the clients or we should know the arrival pattern and service time. The objective of knowing queueing theory is to determine:

- How many channels are required to provide that average given length will not be unreasonable.
- How to schedule arrival so that queue length does not fluctuate too much.
- The cost of queue and cost of service should be beneficial.

Systems Analysis: This is also an operational research technique in which you need to analyze the policies and procedures; qualify and quantify the service in relation to number of hospital beds; treatment of patients in relation to art of care and time spent with each patient and the development of good rapport between doctor and patient.

Diagnostic and Therapeutic Process: Assess each procedure in relation to quality and quantity of test e.g. in an x-ray, you need to see the quality of x-ray, taken, the waiting time for a single x-ray, the type of x-ray, its adequacy in relation to the type of patient and his clinical need, the number of x-rays per day.

Evaluation of Outcome

Assess the outcome of OPD service in relation to patient satisfaction and cost benefit and cost effective analysis.

Patient Satisfaction: Assess by developing a questionnaire about the quality and quantity of service provided. This can also be assessed by interviews of patients, number of complaints.

Employee Satisfaction: Assess the satisfaction of the staff working in OPD by questionnaire so as to improve the service and keep the employees motivated.

Cost Benefit Analysis: Assess the benefits (in term of aid provided for clinical diagnosis) out of any services in terms of cost incurred in providing such a service.

Cost Effective Analysis: Assess each service provided in terms of its cost vis-à-vis its effectiveness to provide the required service e.g. Break Even Analysis can be adopted to study the cost-effectiveness of an equipment, say an x-ray machine.

At the end of this whole process one should be able to qualify and quantify the OPD service provided in any hospital. The analysis of this action plan will help in developing the alternate solutions and select the best course of action (Agarwal, A.K., 2001).

A RESEARCH PLAN FOR STUDYING THE OPERATIONAL EFFICIENCY OF OPDS IN A HOSPITAL

Methodology

The individual carrying out the study for the assessment of OPD services has to develop a methodology, which he/she has to follow during the course of study. One such methodology is given below (Agrawal, M., 1999)

Objectives of Study

It is important to set objectives for study so that it can lead to a fruitful outcome. Some of the objectives are listed below:

- To identify the vision and mission of the hospital.
- To develop a comprehensive profile of the hospital.
- To identify the various OPDs serving the community.
- To identify the OPDs that serve majority of the out-patients and to prepare its comprehensive profile.
- To find out the operational efficiency of the OPDs with respect to response time and service time.
- To assess the level of patient satisfaction on the quality and effectiveness of the OPD services of the hospital.
- To provide suggestions and recommendations for further improving the delivery of effective and efficient health care services at the OPDs.

Research Design

This can be analytical, descriptive or descriptive cum analytical study.

Place of Study

The hospital in which the study will be carried out and the various OPD services it delivers has to be identified.

Duration of the Study

The duration of the study whether it is in weeks, months or years has to be decided. The various activities that will be carried out during the study and the time required to carry out those activities has to be identified.

For instance:

- A study of OPD can be carried out for six months.
- The patient flow and work flow existing in the morning and evening OPDs of the hospital is studied during the first week.
- In the next six weeks the data related to waiting time, service time and response time is collected.

- Patient satisfaction interview data is collected during the same period.
- Each selected speciality is studied for consecutive 2 weeks.

Data Collection Plan

In the first step the OPDs that serve majority of the patients are identified on the basis of last four years. Out-Patient attendance and profiles of the identified OPDs are developed with respect to:

- Layout of the selected OPDs of the hospital.
- Location of the selected OPDs of the hospital.
- Patient attendance in the selected OPDs of the hospital.
- Hierarchy of staff at the selected OPDs of the hospital.
- Profile of patients visiting the selected OPDs of the hospital.
- Public utilities available in the selected OPDs of the hospital

Method of Collection of Information

The method of collection of the above-mentioned information is the following:

- The OPDs are identified on the basis of OP records available in the computer section of the Hospital.
- Information on the location, the layout and the public utilities available in the selected OPDs is collected through on the spot observations at the selected OPDs.
- Information on hierarchy of staff in the selected OPDs is collected by interviewing the staff and subsequently validating it through on the spot observations.
- Information on patient attendance and patient profile is collected from the Out-Patient records.

Information on the following is collected to find out the operational efficiency of the selected OPDs of the hospital:

- Arrival pattern of patients in the morning and evening in selected OPDs of the hospital.
- Work flow at the selected OPDs of the hospital.
- Patient flow at the selected OPDs of the hospital.
- Queue length of patients at the selected OPDs of the hospital.
- Waiting time before availing consultancy services at the selected OPDs of the hospital.

- Response time at the selected OPDs of the hospital.
- Service time at the selected OPDs of the hospital.

The method of collection of information on work flow, arrival pattern, patient flow, waiting time, queue length, response time and service time is the following:

- Work flow and patient flow are understood by interviewing the staff and on the spot observations.
- Arrival pattern of patients is studied for the month of X and Y with the help of OP records.
- Queue length, waiting time, response time and service time are observed. The observations are recorded by randomly selecting each consultant, so that no consultant is missed. The observations are made for each consultant during all working days and different Out-Patient hours.

Information is collected to assess the patient satisfaction through exit interview (the out-patients are interviewed after they have been seen by respective consultant and before they are about to leave the hospital) for the following parameters:

- Assessment of the Reception services
- Behaviour of the OP staff
- Opinion about public utilities available at selected OPDs of the hospital
- Opinion about service quality of the OPDs
- Service charges
- Service time
- Time of waiting before receiving consultancy service of OPDs
- Time spent at the Enquiry Counter
- Time spent at the Registration Counter

Information on the above-mentioned parameters is collected by carrying out a patient satisfaction survey through exit interview with X number of patients (sample size to be determined), visiting the selected OPDs of the hospital. Appropriate questionnaire to be used for interviewing the out-patients has to be developed and tested and if needed be appropriately modified for final interview.

Information collected under different heads enumerated above is to be utilized to find out the operational areas where further improvement is possible.

The operational areas are:

- Arrival of the patient and movement in the hospital
- Patient care
- Public utilities

Identification of the scope of further improving operational management in the selected OPDs is done after analyzing the current state of managing patient/cases in the selected OPDs as per the following plan.

Analysis Plan

The collected data is to be fed in the computer and analyzed by using packages such as

- D Base
- Epi Info
- MS Office

During the analysis various statistical tools are to be used such as:

- Bar graphs
- Cross tables
- Frequency distribution
- Line graphs
  - ✧ The OPDs are identified on the basis of last few years of OP attendance.
  - ✧ All the different OP specialities are arranged in descending order according to total OP attendance and cumulative frequencies are prepared.
  - ✧ OP specialities that cover at-least 70% of OP attendance are selected.
  - ✧ Consultants of each selected OP speciality are arranged in descending order according to total OP attendance and cumulative frequencies are prepared.
  - ✧ Consultants that cover at-least 70% of OP attendance in each OP speciality are selected.
  - ✧ The average queue length, average waiting time, average response time and average service time are calculated for each selected speciality covering all selected consultants.

- The queue length is observed at half an hourly interval by counting the entire OP either waiting to be served or being served. Thus average queue length is calculated by adding all observed queue lengths and dividing by total classes of half an hour interval.
- The waiting time is calculated by subtracting the time at which OP is called to provide service from time when OP submitted OP folder. Thus average waiting time is calculated by adding different waiting time for different OP and divided by total number of observations made.
- Response time is observed by subtracting the service starting time for OP from the time at which OP is called to provide service. Average response time is calculated by adding all observed response time and dividing by number of observations.
- Service time is observed by subtracting the time when service provided to OP ended from the service starting time for OP. The average service time is calculated by adding all observed service time and dividing it by number of observations.
- The responses collected under patient satisfaction interview is analyzed with the help of frequency distribution. Further the relevant cross tables are made and analyzed in order to observe the related factors responsible for the responses given by the patients.

Findings

Identification of OPDs and Profile of selected OPDs

- Identification of OPDs and Consultants
- Location and Layout
- Out-Patient Attendance
- Availability of Public Utilities

Operational Efficiency of the selected OPDs

- Out-patient flow
- Work flow
- Arrival pattern of out-patient
- Queue length, waiting time, response time and service time in selected OPDs of the hospital

Patient Satisfaction Survey

Analysis

The data collected is analyzed based on cross tabulations with different variables and the findings are noted.

Conclusion

A reasonable conclusion based on the findings of the study is drawn by the researcher.

Suggestions

The researcher gives reasonable suggestions based on the findings of the study of the OPDs.

Bibliography

The researcher is supposed to give bibliography at the end of all the reference material used for the study.

CHECKLIST FOR A VISIT TO OPD SERVICES

Evaluation of Structural Criteria

- Location vis-à-vis community and transport facility.
- Site and size of OPD in relation to workload.
- Type of OPD services provided vis-à-vis the needs of the community.
- Adequacy of labour and facilities of space, equipment and stores vis-à-vis the workload in OPD.
- Functional zones of OPD and its adequacy in relation to the OPD patient load.

Evaluation of Process Criteria

- Evaluation of flow of patient traffic keeping in mind the flow concept, holding capacity and lifting capacity.
- Assessment of waiting time by use of various operational research techniques e.g. queuing theory.
- Utilization of man and material by doing a work study and activity sampling.
- Evaluation of policies and procedures of the hospital for OPD with the help of SWOT analysis and system analysis and analysis of records.

- Evaluation of quality and quantity of clinical care to patients in relation to art of care, cure provided, diagnostic accuracy and rapport between doctor and patient, and analysis of records.
- Evaluation of diagnostic and therapeutic procedures both quality and quantity wise.

Evaluation of Outcome Criteria

- Assessment of patient satisfaction by use of questionnaire and interviews, number of complaints and conflicts.
- Assessment of employee satisfaction; grievance procedure for both patients and employees.
- Assessment of outcome of service in terms of cost-benefit and cost effectiveness.

POINTS TO REMEMBER WHILE CARRYING OUT STUDY OF ANY LIVE PROBLEMS IN OPD

- Define the problem
- Carry out critical analysis of the problem
- Possible reasons of the problem
- Collection of facts and figures
- Alternative solutions to the problem
- Selection of best alternative solution with reasons
- Action plan and remedial measures

CONCLUSION

Research is a scientific and systematic search for pertinent information on a specific topic. The main aim of research is to discover answers to questions through the application of scientific procedures. Assessment of OPD services of a hospital is very important and it should be carried out by health care personnel's trained in hospital and health care management, in a scientific way so as to continuously improve the system of delivering OPD health care services to the community. Good OPD services of a hospital will generate *goodwill* of the hospital in the community.

REFERENCES

1. Ackoff, R.L. *The Design of Social Research,* Chicago University Press, Chicago, 1961.
2. Agarwal, A. K. *Practical Manual,* Indira Gandhi National Open University, School of Health Sciences, New Delhi, 2001.
3. Agrawal, M. *Operational Efficiency of the Selected OPDs,* IIHMR, Jaipur, 1999.
4. Harper W. Boyd, Jr., Westfall, R. and Stasch, Stanley F. *Marketing Research-Text and Cases,* Richard D. Irwin INC, A.I.T.B.S. Publishers and Distributors, New Delhi1, 1996.
5. Kothari, C.R. *Research Methodology Methods and Techniques,* Wishwa Prakashan, New Delhi, 1990.
6. Redman, L.V. and Mory, A.V.H. *The Romance of Research,* 1923.
7. Selltiz, C., *et al. Research Methods in Social Sciences,* 1962.
8. Sinha, R.K. and Chattopadhyay, A. *Research Methodology – Basic Concepts and Sampling Techniques,* International Institute For Population Sciences, Mumbai, 2003 (a).
9. Sinha, R.K. and Chattopadhyay, A. *Research Methodology- Research Methods,* International Institute For Population Sciences, Mumbai, 2003 (b).
10. Swarup, K, Guta, P.K. and Mohan, M. *Operations Research,* Sultan Chand & Sons Educational Publishers, New Delhi, 1997.
11. The Advanced Learner's Dictionary of Current English, Oxford, 1952.

5

Problems in Out-Patient (OPD) Services in Hospitals

★ Overview
★ Functions of OPD Services
★ Policies and Procedures in OPD
★ Problems in Out-Patient Services
★ Different Perspectives of Problems in OPD
★ Problems Frequently Seen in OPD Services
★ Where are the Problems in OPD
★ Problems Perceived by the Health Care Staff in OPD
★ Problems Perceived by the Patients and the Community in OPD Services
★ Cause and Effect
★ Problems Related to OPD Procedures
★ Queuing and Waiting Time Problems in OPD Services
★ Problems Related to Laboratory Services in OPD
★ Problems of Physical Facilities in OPD Services
★ Coordination Problems in OPD Services
★ Problems Related to Coordination Among Various Specialities in OPD
★ Problems of Resources in OPD
★ Problems Related to Dispensary in OPD
★ Problems Related to Faith on Doctors
★ Problems Related to the Narrow Perception of Doctors about their Roles in Health Care Services
★ Problems Related to Leadership Qualities Among Hospital Managers
★ Problems of Atmosphere outside the OPD
★ Problems due to Rush of Patients outside OPD

★ Problems due to Improper Management of Medical Record of Patients in the OPD
★ Miscellaneous Considerations that can be taken to Reduce Problems in the OPD Services
★ Summary of Alternate Solutions of Problems of OPD Services
★ Efficiency of OPD Services
★ Method of Improving the Out-Patient Department
★ Conclusion
★ References

OVERVIEW

Out-Patient (OPD) services are the most important service provided by all the hospitals as it provides services to a large number of patients at a low cost. In general hospitals offering primary health care, the same doctor examines all categories of patients while in secondary and tertiary hospitals, patients are examined by competent specialists. Successful and efficient management of OPD can lighten the burden on the in-patient wards. OPD service is one of the rapidly growing services offered by the hospitals. OPD services are being faced with many problems.

Some problems in OPD services are:

- Appointment system jumping
- Long waiting by patients
- Non-availability of test results such as laboratory reports, X-rays, Ultrasonography reports, CT Scan reports etc.
- Interruptions caused by telephones and mobiles in the OPD thus leading to problems in clinical consultations by the doctors.

The hospital is like an industry and must make efforts for maximum consumer's satisfaction and should provide for consumer's oriented service. The problems in OPD services of hospitals are a very important aspect and should be studied in detail so that the problems can be rectified and service quality be continuously improved leading to consumer's satisfaction.

The New Role of a medical practitioner according to WHO (1988) is - "A medical practitioner is a medical doctor able to provide primary health care, either alone in direct contact with the population or as the head of a PHC team delivering at least the eight elements of primary health care".

FUNCTIONS OF OPD SERVICES

The main functions of OPD services are as follows:

- OPD carries out health promotion activities.
- OPD is a route for in-patient admission.
- OPD maintains records and collects data for epidemiological and social research.
- OPD provides after care and medical rehabilitation if necessary after discharge from hospital.
- OPD provides ambulatory and domiciliary treatment to all cases, which can be treated at clinic or at home.
- OPD services are ideal for early diagnosis of any disease with modern techniques and for prophylactic examination.
- OPD participates in various preventive activities such as:
  - ✧ Early reporting of communicable diseases in the community
  - ✧ Health education and nutrition advice
  - ✧ Immunizsation
  - ✧ School health programme
  - ✧ Well baby clinic and ante-natal clinic
- OPD trains medical, nursing and paramedical personnel for delivering health care to the community (Agarwal, A. K., 2001).

POLICIES AND PROCEDURES IN OPD

Because of the interdependence of the staff, facilities and services of the hospital with that of the OPD, it is essential that policies and procedures for each aspect of its functioning should be laid down in writing. A manual should be developed which should be available in the unit at all times for reference of health care personnel.

Policies are guidelines for action in all situations in general.

Procedures aim at putting the policies into practice and in adapting the facilities to the operational needs, and are therefore standardized methods of work.

In order to run the OPD efficiently, policies and procedures should cover both management and technical (professional) aspects of the OPD services.

Due care is required in compilation of the programme of all OPDs. Routinely, a standard programme is prepared on a weekly cycle taking into account the following:

- Availability of medical staff
- Type of accommodation and physical facilities
- Availability of equipment
- Balanced deployment of health care staff

Clear policies and procedures should be understood by all the health care staff appointed in OPD regarding the various aspects of OPD operations (Sakharkar, B.M, 1999). This will help in reducing many of the problems faced by the health care staff deployed in OPD.

PROBLEMS IN OUT-PATIENT SERVICES

A detailed survey of the existing facilities in most hospitals is likely to reveal that the OPD services are not how they are expected to be. Patient overcrowding, poor service and long patient queues, staff and patient dissatisfaction can be noted in varying degree and combinations (Sakharkar, B.M, 1999). Hospital managers should have an in-depth knowledge of the health care system they are managing so that they can tackle any problem faced by the unit. However, before hospital manager can tackle a problem related to the unit he/she has to identify the problem and the factors causing the problem (Vogal, A., 1979).

Any disruption in the smooth functioning of OPD services affects the patients directly or indirectly. There are numerous problems in OPD, one can think of. However, the most common problems encountered in any OPD are as follows:

- Appointment jumping by the patients.
- Long waiting hours at each point of contact of service delivery.
- Non-availability of equipment and supplies in the OPD.
- Non-availability of reports of various investigations due to mismanagement of laboratory and other diagnostic services.
- Non-responsive reception and apathetic staff deployed at the facility.
- Poor rapport or communication between doctors and patients.
- Wild search of speciality OPDs by patients due to improper or absent signage system in the OPD.

The most important cause underlying the problems in OPD service is the *tremendous load* and *increasing demands* for out-patient care by the community, and therefore, an imbalance between demand and resources.

DIFFERENT PERSPECTIVES OF PROBLEMS IN OPD

Problems in OPD services can be looked at from different perspectives such as:

- What are, and where are, the problems?
- Who's view? i.e. problems as seen by the health care staff, the patients, and the community.
- What cause? i.e. a search for the root cause of the problem.
- What effect? i.e. how does it affect the operations of the OPD service.
- How can the problem be solved?

PROBLEMS FREQUENTLY SEEN IN OPD SERVICES

The problems frequently seen in OPD services are grouped below:

- Operations – These are problems related to operational aspects of OPD services. These can be as follows:
  - ✧ Long queues of patient's waiting to be serviced
  - ✧ Queue jumping by the patient's for availing OPD services out of turn
  - ✧ Inadequate service time at various service centres in OPD
  - ✧ Patient's queries not answered by medical staff properly
  - ✧ Punctuality of the medical staff
- Resources – These are problems related to the resources at the disposal of the hospital manager for delivering services in OPD.

These can be as follows:

  - ✧ Inadequacy and incompetence of medical and other support staff
  - ✧ Non-availability of drugs and supplies in OPD

✧ Logistic problems

- Efficiency – These are problems related to the efficiency of the OPD services.
- Physical facilities and layout – These are problems related to the infrastructure of OPD and other physical facilities essential for delivering health care services to the community.
- Quality of care – There may be problems with the quality of care delivered to the patients in OPD.
- Patient and staff satisfaction – There may be problems of satisfaction levels of both the staff and patients. Staff may not be satisfied with the physical facilities provided to him for delivering clinical care to the patient. Patients may not be satisfied with the behaviour of the staff delivering services in OPD.

WHERE ARE THE PROBLEMS IN OPD

Key areas where problems in OPD operations can be faced are:

- Reception and Enquiry
- Registration procedures
- Patient Flow
- Clinics
- Laboratory counter
- Injection room
- Dressing room
- Dispensary

PROBLEMS PERCEIVED BY THE HEALTH CARE STAFF IN OPD

Problems perceived by the health care staff delivering services in OPD are likely to be different from those perceived by the patients and the community, although some times there may be some overlap. The staff may complain of:

- Shortage of manpower
- Frequent breakdowns and non-availability of equipment
- Drugs and supplies out of stock
- Too many patient

PROBLEMS PERCEIVED BY THE PATIENTS AND THE COMMUNITY IN OPD SERVICES

Problems perceived by the patients and the community are as follows:

- Long queues
- Long waiting time
- Inadequate service time
- Staff not being courteous
- Unpunctuality of staff

CAUSE AND EFFECT

It is difficult to differentiate between cause and effect, but the distinction is important. Remedial measures for OPD problems must be directed to the root cause of the problem. Many problems may have several causes, and one cause may have many effects.

PROBLEMS RELATED TO OPD PROCEDURES

It is frequently observed that there are delays and wastage of time of patients attending OPD services of the hospitals. A number of patients complained that they have to waste a lot of time in waiting for their turn in the OPD. They at times have to wait for 2-3 hours to see the doctor concerned and to avail the services of the OPD. The doctors, on the contrary, complain that patients visit most of the hospitals again and again without making use of the earlier medical records. Some patients complain that the doctors examine the VIP patients in preference to other patients (Goel, S.L. and Kumar, 2004).

Suggestions

- There is a need for streamlining the procedures in OPD so that the delay can be avoided.
- The patients at the time of registration at the registration counter may be advised by the person manning the counter about the probable time of his turn, this will help the patient in chalking out his schedule.
- The patients from the village may be given preference at the OPD for examination and consultation so that they can go

back to their village after examination and consultation by the doctor and thus may not unnecessarily crowd the hospital premises.

QUEUING AND WAITING TIME PROBLEMS IN OPD SERVICES

OPD services of the majority of the hospitals have queuing and waiting time problems.

Factors affecting the service of an OPD are the following (Sakharkar, B.M, 1999):

- *Arrival pattern,* or input rate, of patients at the central waiting room/lounge
- *Input and output rates* at various clinics and other supportive services units of OPD
- *Service time* at various clinics of OPD
- *Queue lengths* at waiting rooms of clinics of OPD

The above-mentioned factors are interdependent. Queue lengths and waiting time at the central waiting room/lounge are related to the input rate at the waiting room and output rate at the doctors' clinics. The problem is a result of a large number of patients arriving early, coupled with late start of clinics in OPD.

Suggestions

Queuing and waiting line problems can be managed in the following manner.

Appointment System: After the first visit, the patients are given the date and time for their next visit. This ensures greater involvement of doctors in making as well as keeping appointments. The doctor must keep a few appointments vacant to serve the serious patients who may have to be attended out of turn.

Principles of Appointment System are as follows:

- The rate of calling patients to the clinic by appointment should match the particular doctor's rate of dealing with them.
- The appointment system should also take into consideration the net unpunctuality of both patients and doctor and the average extent of nonattendance by patients.
- If the net average increase or decrease in attendance is ca-

tered for in the appointment system, then the effects on waiting times of irregularities in attendance can be very slight when averaged over a large number of clinics.

Types of Appointment System

Individual Appointments System - The appointment at a particular time is for individual patients. The physician may at time find himself or herself idle

Block Appointment System - The appointment at a particular time is for a block of patients. It is intended to provide a pool of patients so that the physician will at no time find himself or herself idle

Advantages of staggering of the appointment times are:

- Can decongest the crowd
- Shorten the queues
- Lessen unnecessary waiting item of the patients

Disadvantages of Appointment System are:

- Invariably, some patients fail to attend and others arrive without appointment.
- The system leads to long waiting lines for a majority of the patients.
- Smart patients try to outwit the system by arriving late.

Filter Clinics: It is observed that all patients visiting the OPD services of hospitals do not require care by specialists. A large majority of diseases can be managed at the level of non specialist general duty doctors, filter clinics, clinically manned by such doctors are able to relieve congestion on speciality clinics of the hospitals. Filter clinics should be integral parts of the hospital's OPD.

Satellite Clinics: Satellite clinics are located away from the main hospital OPD, to serve defined sections of populations, but have links with the main hospital. These clinics can be clinically managed entirely by general duty doctors, but with arrangements for referral of the patients to the hospitals specialist out-patient clinics as well as by occasional consultation visits to satellite clinic by specialists of the main OPD services of the hospitals.

Selective Service Charge: High demand of OPD services in government and charity hospitals may be discouraged by a high selective service charge to those patients who come directly to the specialty clinics without having passed through a filter clinic or satellite clinic, or without any type of referral from any other physician who is providing services separately from the hospital. If the peoples economic condition is good this method will not yield good results and may be counterproductive for the OPD services of the hospital.

Starting OPD in Time and Prolonging OPD Timings: It is essential that unpunctuality in OPD must be avoided at all costs by the health care staff of the OPD services. The staff must start the clinics as per the declared timings and must always strictly follow these timings. If patients know that the OPD starts at 10 AM, so the doctor and staff should be in position to see the first patient at 10 AM.

By prolonging the OPD timings till late afternoon or evening with a suitable break for the staff would enable a larger number of patients to be clinically dealt with. Some hospitals experimented to start evening OPD services but these have not produced the desired effect. However, prolonging the existing OPD timings till evening appears to have a better chance of success than starting evening OPD. The extended timings of the OPD must be matched by all the supportive services of the OPD like laboratory and dispensary etc.

PROBLEMS RELATED TO LABORATORY SERVICES IN OPD

It has been frequently observed that the laboratory services in OPDs are inadequate and this results in unnecessary harassment of the consumer's of the OPD services of the hospitals. A large number of the patients after examination by doctors in OPD are advised various tests such as urine test, blood test (TLC, DLC, ESR, etc), stool examination (routine, microscopic for ova, cyst, worms, occult blood etc.), sputum examination, etc. Patients have to stand in long queues in laboratory services for every test and this consumes a lot of time. Due to non-functional equipment in many hospitals, patients have to get these tests done at other hospitals at a very high cost. Patients even feel that doctors in the hospitals are in collusion with the clinics outside and thus deliberately refer the patients to these clinics. The results of these tests generally do not move automatically to the file of the patient, rather the patient or his relatives have to collect the results of these tests. The doctors examine these results after 3-4 days when his turn comes next time. There is also a lot of problem relating to the quality of these tests. If the tests are not of good quality then the results may not be up to the mark and this may lead to wrong diagnosis and thus clinical management of the disease may be affected.

Suggestions

- There is a need of rejuvenating the laboratory services in hospitals.
- It is essential to manage laboratory services efficiently because the prescription of drugs by the doctors is based on the results of the tests.
- Quality of laboratory tests should be good.
- The results of the tests should be made available by evening the same day (as far as possible) so that most of the patients coming from out-stations can leave to their villages and avoid the high living cost of the city life.

PROBLEMS OF PHYSICAL FACILITIES IN OPD SERVICES

There may be various physical facilities problems in OPD services of the hospital such as insufficient waiting space, toilets, drinking water facilities and uncomfortable seating arrangement for patients and their attendant in OPD. Accurate finding of the problems would require in-depth study of each problem by the professionally trained hospital manager.

Methods of Study

- Study of flow charts
- Work study, *viz.* time and motion study, method study, an activity sampling

This will help in determining appropriate solutions to the problems of OPD services.

Suggestions

The hospital management should do the following in order to reduce physical facilities problems in OPD services:

- Adequate number of examination cubicles for each doctor should be provided in the OPD of the hospital.

- Adequate toilets in OPD should be there.
- Clean drinking water in OPD should be there.
- Comfortable seating arrangement in OPD should be there.
- Inadequacies in the structure of the OPD services hampering smooth flow of patients and creating bottlenecks can often be rectified by relatively minor modifications such as adding a door or window, demolishing a wall, shifting a wash basin or tap, partitioning a room into cubicles, widening a passage and so on and so forth.
- Sufficient waiting spaces, both at the central waiting area and at the clinic must be provided for patients and their attendants attending the OPD.

COORDINATION PROBLEMS IN OPD SERVICES

It is frequently observed that there are coordination problems in day-to-day activities of OPD services in the hospitals since many activities are simultaneously occurring within a short span of 4 to 5 hours in busy OPD services.

It has been noted that in many public hospitals, it is not possible for a physician or a group of the physicians to effectively control and coordinate the day-to-day activities of the OPD services.

It has also been found by researchers that as little as 7 per cent of qualified nursing staff time is found to be spent on nursing work.

Suggestions

- The basic requirement in OPD services is coordination and control of all the OPD operations, which can be achieved by unity of command by one person over all the OPD operations.
- The responsibility for the day-to-day functioning and coordination of staff and facilities should, be of an official who is directly responsible to the chief administrator of the hospital, and who must have authority to participate in the policy decisions in that capacity. OPD administrator should have full status of department head.
- It is debatable that whether the physician administrator having responsibility for the overall functioning and coordina-

tion of the departmental should take clinics himself. The size and complexity of the OPD would determine this. In a large OPD where the physician-administrator has this overall responsibility he or she should not take any clinics himself or herself.

- A high degree of collaboration between the various clinics, supportive services and other elements of OPD could be achieved by the OPD administrator by the following:
  - ✧ Daily rounds of the facility
  - ✧ Continuous monitoring of the facility
  - ✧ Informal discussions with medical and other staff of the facility
  - ✧ Periodical meetings with medical staff of the facility
  - ✧ Coordination through medico administrative committees of the facility framed by hospital management
- Preparation of a management check-list for OPD services, phrased as question to a patient can be developed by the management of each hospital taking into account the peculiarities of each hospital.
- In each OPD, there should be a sister incharge who devotes her time mainly to the supervision and coordination of the work of nursing, auxiliary and paramedical workers deployed in OPD clinics.

PROBLEMS RELATED TO COORDINATION AMONG VARIOUS SPECIALITIES IN OPD

There is lack of coordination among various specialities in the OPD services. It has been generally observed that patients visiting one speciality are referred to other facilities as well for cross-reference and consultation. This is a time consuming process and demoralises the patients as well.

Suggestions

- There is a need of integrating the efforts of the specialists.
- It is suggested that such patients may be examined by a board of specialists once a week so that they are examined from all the angles before the clinical management of the patient is initiated.

PROBLEMS OF RESOURCES IN OPD

There may be resources problems in OPD services of the hospitals, which are at the disposal of hospital manager for the delivery of efficient OPD services to the community. The resources include *men, materials* and *money.*

Suggestions

- In order to have proper resource utilization one has to have a well-planned and coordinated deployment of men, materials and money in OPD services.
- Dearth of resources in OPD services is often relative. An apparent shortage of staff may reflect faulty deployment of available staff by the OPD coordinator. Appropriate remedial measures to be taken to rectify the staff deployment problem.
- Materials and supplies required to meet the functions of the OPD services need to be made continuously available.
- The allotment of resources must meet the fluctuating requirements of the OPD services.
- Methods to reduce costs and improve efficiency need to be continuously monitored, especially in the use of drugs, radiographic films, and other consumable items of general surgical and medical use.
- Prescription of commonly used drugs under many brand names, and pre packing of drugs for issue through dispensary is an attempt in cost reduction, variety reduction, and waste reduction.

PROBLEMS RELATED TO DISPENSARY IN OPD

It is frequently observed that there is non-availability of medicines of various diseases in the dispensary of OPD services. This is because of low budget allocated to the dispensary and pilferage of medicines from the dispensary. Medicines supplied from the dispensary are at times of inferior quality and this affects the outcome of clinical management of the patient. This spreads the poor image of the working of the hospitals.

Suggestions

- There is a need ensuring the supply of right quality medicine to the patients. This can be achieved by procuring drugs from reputed and approved manufacturers and suppliers.

- Hospital management should keep an eye on the dispensary so as to ensure that the right drug and quality drug is being supplied to the patients.
- List of medicines available at the dispensary, their manufacturers and suppliers must be displayed outside the dispensary so that patients can check and be satisfied.

PROBLEMS RELATED TO FAITH ON DOCTORS

It is frequently observed that people complain that the doctors in government/semi-government hospitals do not bother much about the patients and that is why there is mushroom growth of private health care practitioners or the coming up of a large number of nursing homes and private hospitals. It is in contravention to the Directive Principles of the State Policy enshrined in the Constitution of India that the Government would ensure the provisions of decent health care for all at a cost that the people can afford. Moreover, behaviour of the doctors is rude and thus act as repellant to the patients visiting the OPD.

Suggestions

- There is a need of educating the people about their rights *vis-a-vis* the hospitals so that the services available in the hospitals are utilized efficiently.
- There is a need of creating a good public opinion.
- Programmes should be organized for doctors in order to generate awareness among them about the importance of human relations.

PROBLEMS RELATED TO THE NARROW PERCEPTION OF DOCTORS ABOUT THEIR ROLES IN HEALTH CARE SERVICES

It is frequently observed that most of the doctors think that their job is simply to examine the visiting patients and prescribe treatment to them. This is a negative approach. The doctors in OPD must utilize this opportunity to act as health and medical leaders to bring about revolution in the health status of the people of the catchment area of the hospital.

Suggestions

- There is a need of broadening the vision and functions of the doctors.
- The various functions and activities of doctors that they should be made aware of are as follows:
  - ✧ As a Physician - treatment of patients, promotion of health at community and individual levels, prevention of diseases and accidents and rehabilitation.
  - ✧ As an Educator – of oneself, health personnel, patients and the community.
  - ✧ As a Manager – to maintain good and harmonious relationship with referral services, communities and their representatives, development of research activities and to be a leader of teams of health care personnel.
  - ✧ As an Agent of socio-economic development – to participate in community development activities.

These functions and activities should be complemented, adapted and detailed further, as needed, to cope with local situations of the region.

PROBLEMS RELATED TO LEADERSHIP QUALITIES AMONG HOSPITAL MANAGERS

It is frequently observed that Chief Medical Officers (CMOs), Medical Superintendents, Deputy Medical Superintendents, Administrators and other managers do not make use of the talent available in the doctors in a right way. They can get more work done out of them if they are properly motivated. An efficient OPD generates a positive opinion about the hospital among the community. It is observed that hospital managers lack proper leadership qualities and as result they are not able to manage teams in a proper way and thus the potential of the team remains under utilized.

Suggestions

- There is a need to develop leadership Qualities among Hospital Managers.
- The qualities in health leaders, must be taken up by the hospital managers.

- Hospital managers need to have strong commitment, ability to communicate, courage to take risks and make bold decisions
- Hospital mangers should have faith in the people's potentials as it will make the team more confident and they will be able to deliver high quality OPD services to the community.
- There is need to generate awareness among Hospital Managers that if the team they are leading is being properly motivated, counseled then they will be able to deliver high quality, efficient and effective health care in the OPD.
- Workshops, seminars and training programmes should be organized for the Hospital Managers to upgrade their leadership qualities.
- Hospital Managers should be made aware of that the leader grows more and lasts longer by placing the well-being of all above the well-being of self alone.
- Hospital managers should be made aware of different leadership styles for managing an organization.

PROBLEMS OF ATMOSPHERE OUTSIDE THE OPD

It is frequently observed that the atmosphere outside the OPD is dull and awful. Majority of the patients and their relatives who wait outside the OPDs feel insecure. The patients and their relatives are afraid of the consequences of the diseases for which they have reported to the unit. Patients suffering from different diseases congregate at the same place and make the situation still more serious and increase the chances of spread of cross infection among patients if the atmosphere outside OPD is not hygienic. The OPD in hospitals are not given due attention and sanitary conditions most of the times don't exist there. The OPD are not properly decorated in most of the hospitals.

Suggestions

- It is suggested that the hospital management must decorate the waiting lounges with meaningful literature outside the OPDs.
- Hospital management should use the opportunity for

providing health-education to patients and their attendants reporting to the OPD.

- The colours of the walls of waiting lounges, the intensity of light, the type of lights etc. should be scientifically decided based on the recommendations of the hospital architect and consultants so that a comfortable environment is created in the OPDs.
- Hygienic conditions should be maintained by the sanitary staff in OPD.

PROBLEMS DUE TO RUSH OF PATIENTS OUTSIDE OPD

It has been frequently observed that the OPD are overcrowded and it becomes very difficult for the doctors to examine patients properly. This results into superficial checkups done hurriedly by the doctors. There are some OPDs where doctors do not get even the minimum number of patients for practicing medicine.

Suggestions

- It is suggested that statistics may be collected for 2-3 years and health care personnel may be appointed according to the findings of the study so that the decent medical care may be made available to all reporting for availing health care services at the OPD.
- If there is high disease incidence of any disease in the region then the number of OPD services offering service for the management of that disease must be more.
- Some norm must be worked out for appointment of medical staff in order to optimize the use of qualified personnel in delivering efficient health care services at the OPD.
- Doctors must be appointed according to the need of the hospital depending upon their speciality and the disease load of certain diseases existing in the community

PROBLEMS DUE TO IMPROPER MANAGEMENT OF MEDICAL RECORD OF PATIENTS IN THE OPD

It is frequently observed that treating doctors advice frequent medical check-ups for their patients. No medical records of patients are maintained for various medical check-ups done from time to time.

Suggestions

It is suggested that people reporting to OPD should be provided with permanent pass-books which can keep a chronological record of the health of the individuals. This can help the doctors in prescribing right medicine to the patient.

Computerized medical records of patients reporting to OPDs must also be generated in addition to the customary medical records so that information about the patients may also be available on line to doctors. This will also reduce the service time at the various service centres at the OPD.

There is a need of introducing modern management methods of maintaining medical records of patients so that quality of service in OPD is improved and the OPD becomes more efficient.

MISCELLANEOUS CONSIDERATIONS THAT CAN BE TAKEN TO REDUCE PROBLEMS IN THE OPD SERVICES

- At the OPD records and registration, common problems frequently seen are delay in locating and retrieval of medical records due to faulty filing, numbering and storage. At present many small hospitals do not have the services of medical record librarians, At least one medical record librarian having appropriate training in management of medical records in even the smallest hospital should be available, who can then train the other paramedical staff in the OPD to maintain OPD records under his or her overall supervision and guidance.
- Sufficient space and filing racks for storage of medical records should be ensured, with identification numbers on each rack and shelf. Numbering of cards by a hand-operated machine should be introduced to obviate misinterpreting of numbers, which is one of the most common reason of confusion in a busy OPD.
- Arrangement to position the records of patients by appointment on the desks of concerned doctors in advance must be organized by the OPD administrator.

- Use of cards of different colours could also be considered for different speciality clinics in the OPD to avoid confusions.
- During busy hours at the enquiry and registration there may be a need to supplement the services with additional staff. It is observed that some voluntary groups offer their services in large towns and cities. The hospital should have the services of at least one medical social worker in the OPD who can help in many ways such as help to arrange for indigent patients drugs not stocked by the hospital, arrange help for the physically handicapped and otherwise incapacitated patients in going about the OPD services.
- The working of the OPD supportive services, central injection room, specimen collection centre, pharmacy and radio diagnosis also need to be continuously monitored by the OPD administrator.
- In the injection room, sufficient availability of syringes and needles should be ensured by the OPD administrator.
- At the specimen collection centre, facilities and staff to draw blood samples and for collecting urine and stool samples should be adequate depending on the requirements.
- Laboratory investigation reports should be made promptly and easily available with an in-built system of prompt distribution of reports to specialists of OPD.
- Insufficient number of counters and short supply of drugs are the two chief problems in Dispensary. It should be ensured that sufficient number of pharmacists should be available to man all counters during the busiest hours of OPD services.
- Hospital should develop a reasonable standard of efficiency in the utilization of staff and facilities in the out-patient department. Laying down policies and procedures for various aspects of OPD operation should help in many cases. The policies and procedures should be made known to staff deployed at the facility, and those which concern to patients should be made known to them in brief terms, by notices displayed at appropriate places and time. The policies should cover overall operational, administrative and technical aspects of OPD functioning.
- Many problems may be beyond solution by the OPD administrator and would require decision and support from the

hospital's top management or other higher authority, there is always scope for improving OPD operations in most hospitals. Constant efforts should be made to improve things in OPD by:

- ✧ Simplification
- ✧ Combination
- ✧ Improved organization
- ✧ Delegation of authority and responsibility
- ✧ Discipline
- ✧ Task allocations and job description for various categories of health care staff
- ✧ Communication
- ✧ Improved motivation of the health care staff

- Due to an imbalance between demand and available resources, the long-term solution to the problems caused by sheer numbers can only be solved by providing more OPD services.
- The only short-term solution to the present situation is to try for increased efficiency. This in turn requires reconsideration of the established operational policies and management procedures.
- Consideration of the long-term solution must also be taken up simultaneously by the hospital management.

SUMMARY OF ALTERNATE SOLUTIONS OF PROBLEMS OF OPD SERVICES

On analysis of various problems in OPD services, one shall find that the following could be the alternate solutions to the problems.

The most common alternate solutions are:

- 24 hrs registration system to fix appointments for old cases and accommodating emergency cases as early as possible, to reduce waiting time in OPD.
- Appointment system in OPD to reduce the waiting time of patients.
- Efficient department of hospital management for day to day redressal of OPD problems.

- **Filter Clinics**: Clinics in the ground floor with junior duty doctors so that minor diseases like cough, cold can be treated and sent back so that they do not overcrowd the speciality OPD of the hospital.
- **Satellite Clinic**: Community outreach clinics of the hospital will reduce the OPD load in the main hospital OPD and the Community will get special care at its door steps.
- Selective attachment of services e.g. having neurosurgery and neurology OPD close by because many of the neurosurgery cases need neurology assessment too. This will lead to a reduction in the patient traffic in other OPD areas.
- Separate general and emergency OPD, to attend the serious cases on priority.
- Starting the OPD in time to reduce the waiting time and prolonging OPD time with another shift of doctors to provide services to maximum number of patients.
- Sufficient waiting area with adequate resources to cater the load.
- Sufficient space for future expansion OPD services.
- Appropriate signage system to be used in order to reduce identification problems of OPDs by the patients.

EFFICIENCY OF OPD SERVICES

The efficiency of OPD services is very important and the OPD administrator has to take care that the services delivered by OPD to the community are efficient and of high quality. The various aspects need to be known by OPD administrator for providing quality OPD services are as follows:

- OPD services of hospital can be the starting point of quality of medical care being delivered by the hospital.
- Good OPD services can reduce the load on in-patient department of the hospital. It can optimize the use of supporting services like Radiology, Pathology, c1inical laboratories and other diagnostic facilities.
- The hour and timing of OPD services, staff deployed in the OPD to deal with the load of patient, queuing time are the operational aspects which should be gathered continuously and action ensured with a view to improve the quality of service delivered at the unit.

- Medical Record Keeping and ensuring continuity of treatment on longitudinal basis should be ensured even in OPD, as it cuts short the cost of treatment, doctor's time and leads to better quality of service.
- The other indices for measuring the quality of services of a hospital are: cure rate, improved cases rate, death rate, unit-wise and department-wise can be monitored on regular basis with frequency determined suitably. These serve as self-assessment of the procedures and interventions undertaken by the respective department.
- Post-operative complication and death rate in surgical departments can be a pointer towards needed introspection of the department [Goel, S.L. and Kumar, R., 2004 (a)]

METHOD OF IMPROVING THE OUT-PATIENT DEPARTMENT

The various methods that can be used for improving the OPD are enumerated below:

- Analyze the diagnoses of the patients attending the OPD, find their six most common diseases.
- Determine the simplest, cheapest and most effective routine for treating these diseases. Cut out any unnecessary treatments.
- Teach auxiliaries how to diagnose and treat these diseases.
- Pay particular attention to more serious conditions, which they must learn to distinguish from them.
- Provide the relevant equipment, rubber stamps, prepacked drugs, stationery, etc., and especially enough of the simple things like dressing forceps.
- Trace the flow of the patients through the building of the OPD. Can this be rationalized by simple works services such as the alteration of doors, the provision of hatches, etc.?
- Examine the queues that form in OPD. What is the cause of the delays? Can these be removed by altering the disposition of staff, providing more auxiliaries, reducing unnecessary clerical work or providing additional apparatus?
- Where relevant let the auxiliaries listen in on your

consultations with the referred cases, so that they may learn continually and continuously upgrade their technical skills.

- Whatever the success of the above measures, some patients are probably still going to spend a long time waiting. Try to see that they wait in reasonable comfort in the OPD waiting areas (Kumar, A., 2000).

CONCLUSION

Out-Patient (OPD) Services are the most important service provided by all the hospitals as it provides services to a large number of patients at a low cost. A detailed survey of the existing facilities in most hospitals is likely to reveal that the OPD services are not how they are expected to be. Patient overcrowding, poor service and long patient queues, staff and patient dissatisfaction can be noted in varying degree and combinations. The most important cause underlying the problems in OPD service is the tremendous load and increasing demands for out-patient care by the community, and therefore, an imbalance between demand and resources. Hospital management should take appropriate steps to find relevant solutions to the problems of OPD services so that the unit continuously improves and provides efficient quality health care to the community.

REFERENCES

1. Agarwal, A. K. *Practical Manual,* Indira Gandhi National Open University, School of Health Sciences, New Delhi, 2001.
2. Goel, S.L. and Kumar, R. *Hospital Core Services-Hospital Administration in the 21st Century,* Deep and Deep Publications Pvt. Ltd., New Delhi, 2004.
3. Goel, S.L. and Kumar, R. *Hospital Supportive Services-Hospital Administration in the 21st Century,* Deep and Deep Publications Pvt. Ltd., New Delhi, 2004 (a).
4. Kumar, A. *Encyclopaedia of Hospital Administration and Development,* Vol.2, Institute For Sustainable Development Lucknow & Anmol Publications Pvt. Ltd., New Delhi, 2000.
5. Sakharkar, B.M. *Principles of Hospital Administration and Planning,* Jaypee Brothers Medical Publishers (P) Ltd., New Delhi, 1999.
6. Vogal, A. *Approaches to Planning and Design of Health-Care Facilities in Developing Areas,* WHO, Geneva, II, 1979.
7. WHO *Issue of World Health Organization,* 1988.

Annexure 1

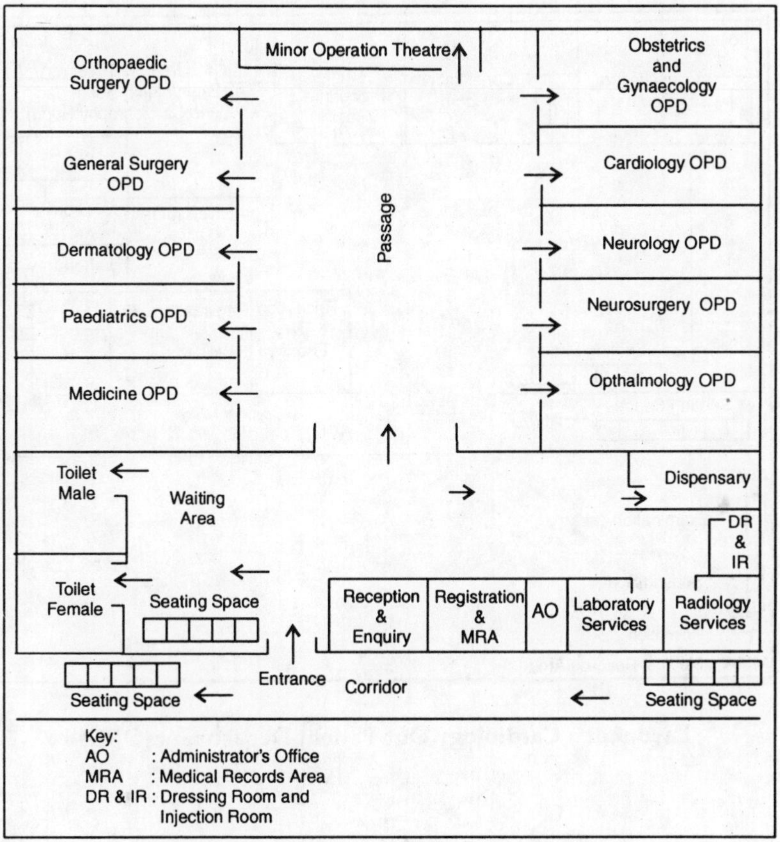

Layout of an Out-Patient Department (OPD)

Annexure 2

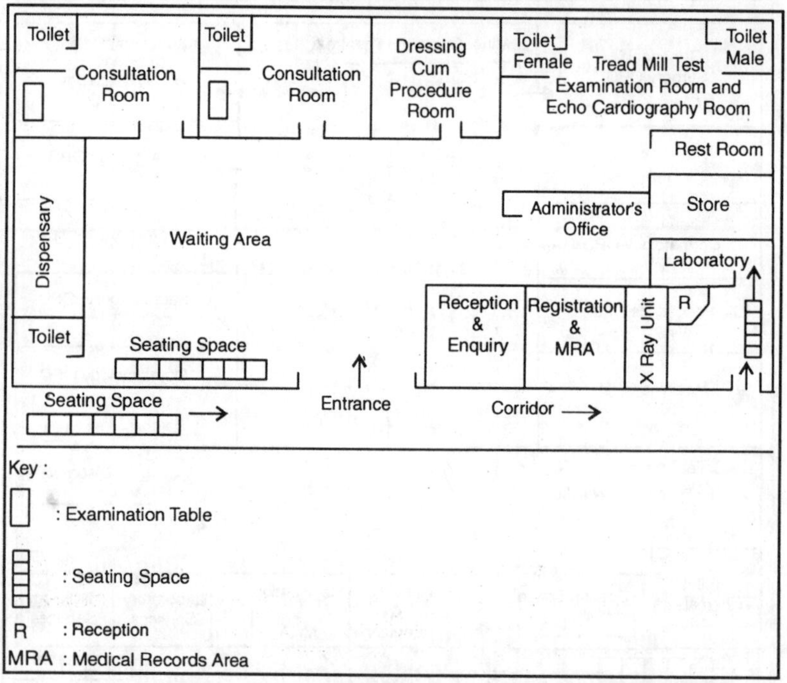

Layout of a Cardiology Out-Patient Department (OPD)

Annexure 3

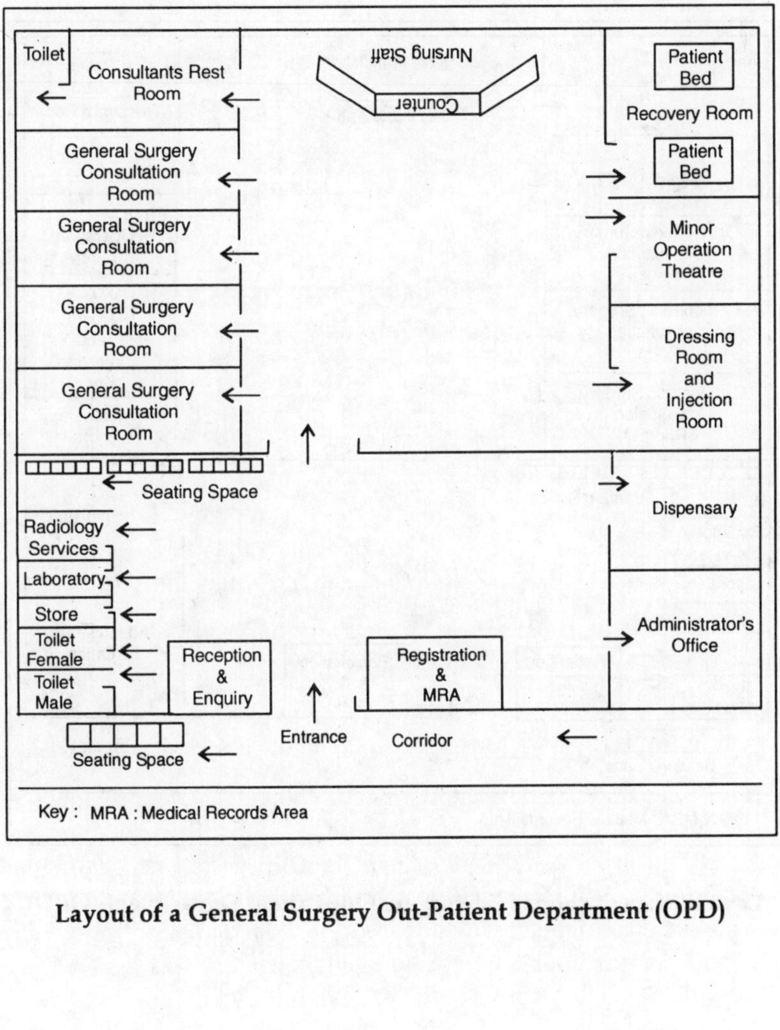

Layout of a General Surgery Out-Patient Department (OPD)

Annexure 4

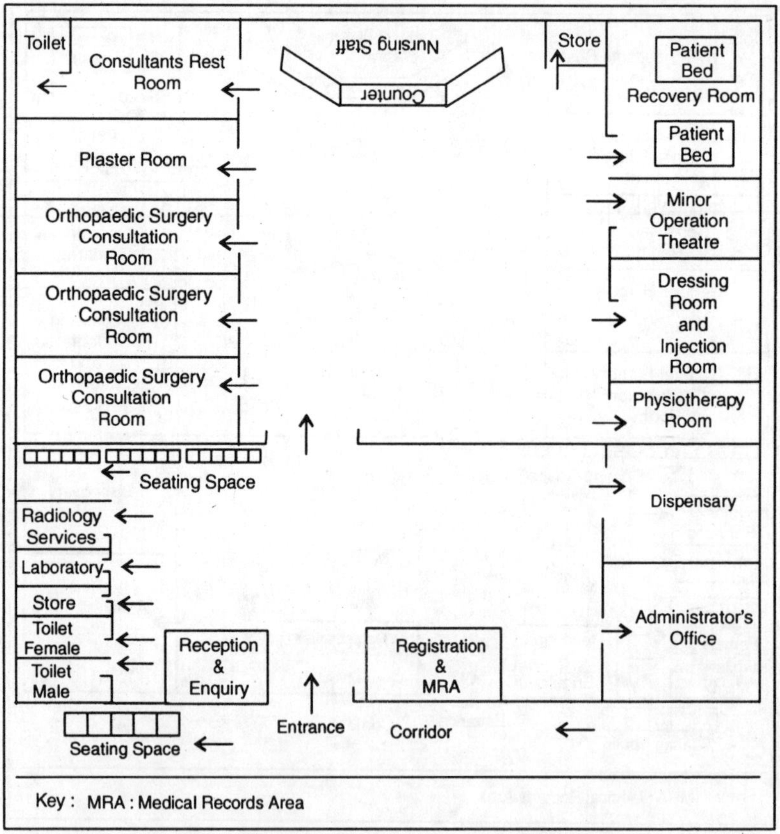

Layout of an Orthopaedic Surgery Out-Patient Department (OPD)

Annexure 5

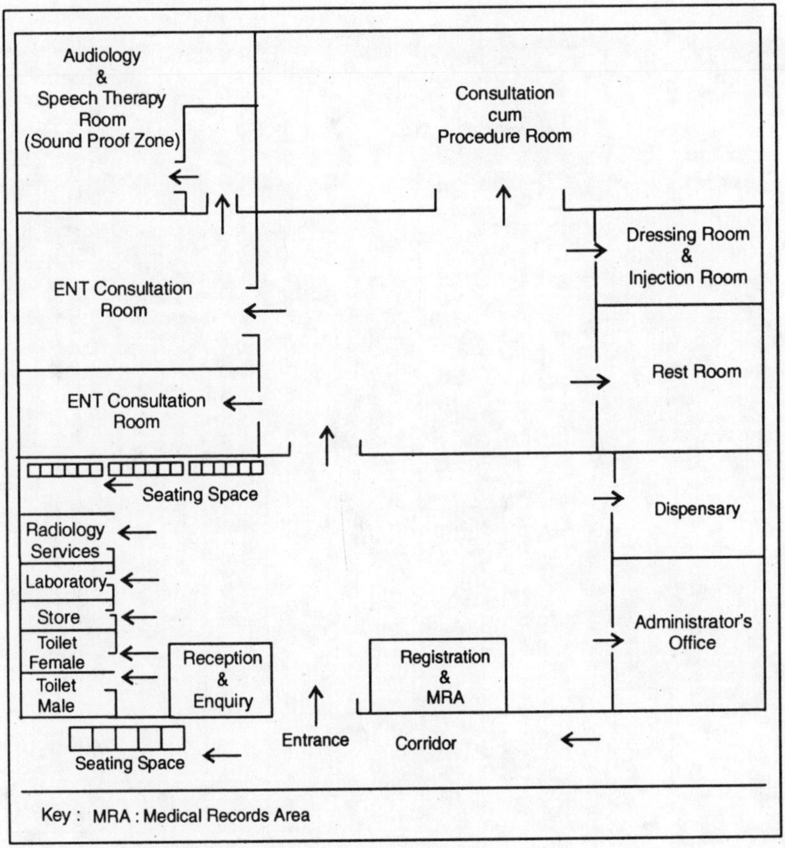

Layout of an ENT Out-Patient Department (OPD)